PREGNANCY DIET PLAN

(2021 EDITION)

EASY GUIDE FOR A PREGNANCY NUTRITION AND A FIT CHILDBIRTH

Angela Poshi

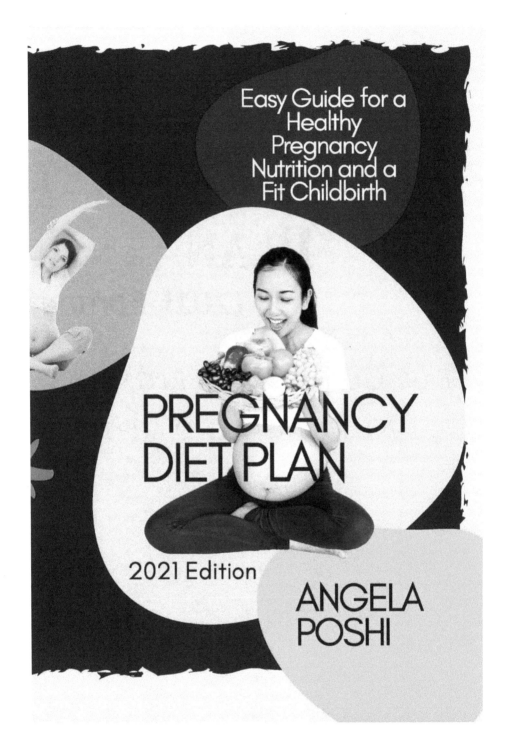

Easy Guide for a Healthy Pregnancy Nutrition and a Fit Childbirth

PREGNANCY DIET PLAN

2021 Edition

ANGELA POSHI

PREGNANCY DIET PLAN

PLAN

(2021 EDITION)

EASY GUIDE FOR A PREGNANCY NUTRITION AND A FIT CHILDBIRTH

Angela Poshi

for any hardship or damages that may befall them after undertaking information described herein.

Additionally, the information in the following pages is intended only for informational purposes and should thus be thought of as universal. As befitting its nature, it is presented without assurance regarding its prolonged validity or interim quality. Trademarks that are mentioned are done without written consent and can in no way be considered an endorsement from the trademark holder.

Introduction

FINDING OUT YOU ARE PREGNANT FOR THE FIRST TIME, OR INDEED THE SECOND, THIRD, OR FOURTH TIMES, CAN BRING ON A MYRIAD OF EMOTIONS: JOY, EXCITEMENT, RETICENCE, FEAR, AWE, CURIOSITY, AND, OF COURSE, ANXIETY. THESE FEELINGS ARE ENTIRELY NATURAL, AS IS THE NEED FOR ADVICE. IN THE PAST, SOCIETIES WITH LARGE FAMILIES AND DIFFERENT SOCIAL STRUCTURES CREATED A NETWORK OF SISTERLY SUPPORT TO HELP AND INFORM WOMEN ABOUT ALL MATTERS PREGNANCY RELATED. BY CONTRAST, TODAY WE MAY TALK ABOUT OUR PREGNANCY TO ONLY A HANDFUL OF FAMILY MEMBERS AND GIRLFRIENDS; AND TO OUR OBSTETRICIAN OR MIDWIFE EVERY COUPLE OF WEEKS.

OFTEN, OUR FIRST STEP IS TO PERFORM AN INTERNET SEARCH. HERE THERE IS AN ABUNDANCE OF INFORMATION (AND MISINFORMATION), AND ANECDOTES OF THE PREGNANCY AND CHILDBIRTH EXPERIENCES OF OTHER PARENTS—INCLUDING THOSE WHAT IS LIKELY TO OCCUR DURING YOUR PREGNANCY, FROM PROCEDURES AND ULTRASOUNDS TO BIRTH

PLANS AND LABOR TECHNIQUES. YOU WILL LEARN ABOUT NUTRITION AND EXERCISE, AND HOW TO KEEP HEALTHY, AS WELL AS THE BIOLOGICAL CHANGES TAKING PLACE IN YOUR BODY AND YOUR BABY'S. THERE ARE ALSO SECTIONS ON CLOTHES TO BUY TO ACCOMMODATE YOUR INCREASINGLY LARGE BELLY, AND ALSO WHAT TO BUY TO PREPARE FOR YOUR NEW ARRIVAL. YOU'LL FIND GUIDANCE ON ALL CONCERNS FROM COMMON COMPLAINTS DURING THE FIRST TRIMESTER TO TAKING CARE OF YOUR NEWBORN. WHEN THE TIME COMES TO SEEK ADVICE FROM YOUR OWN OBSTETRICIAN, WE HAVE ASKED YOU TO DO SO.

THE STORY OF THE BEGINNINGS OF YOUR BABY'S LIFE IS TOLD IN A VISUALLY BEAUTIFUL, EASY-TO-READ, AND FACTUALLY THAT ARE UNUSUALLY GOOD OR UNUSUALLY DISAPPOINTING. SOMETIMES SEARCH RESULTS ARE INFORMATIVE BUT TOO OFTEN THEY CAN BE CONFUSING AND LEAD TO FURTHER ANXIETY ABOUT OUR OWN EXPERIENCE.

PREGNANCY COMES WITH A BEWILDERING ARRAY OF ADVICE ON WHAT YOU SHOULD AND SHOULDN'T DO TO KEEP YOU AND YOUR BABY HEALTHY.

A HEALTHY DIET IS COMPRISED OF THE RIGHT BALANCE OF NUTRITIOUS FOODS FROM SEVERAL MAIN FOOD GROUPS: PROTEIN, FRUIT, VEGETABLES, UNREFINED CARBOHYDRATES, AND HEALTHY FATS. YOU SHOULD EAT FOODS FROM THESE GROUPS IN THEIR MOST NATURAL, UNPROCESSED STATE TO RECEIVE THE MAXIMUM NUMBER OF NUTRIENTS.

THE CHANGES TO YOUR BODY IN PREGNANCY IMPACT MANY ASPECTS OF LIFE, FROM YOUR RELATIONSHIP WITH YOUR PARTNER TO YOUR ABILITY TO STAY COMFORTABLE AND SLEEP, TO MAKING TRAVEL ARRANGEMENTS. IN ADDITION TO THESE PRACTICAL MATTERS, THIS CHAPTER ALSO EXPLORES THE MANY PHYSICAL AND EMOTIONAL CHANGES PREGNANCY BRINGS, AND LOOKS AT SOME OF THE COMMON COMPLAINTS AND COMPLICATIONS OF PREGNANCY AND HOW TO MANAGE THEM.

TO ALL THOSE CONTEMPLATING PREGNANCY, OR WHO ARE ALREADY PREGNANT, I HOPE YOU WILL FIND THAT THIS FASCINATING BOOK HELPS YOU UNDERSTAND AND ENJOY THE VERY BEGINNING OF YOUR BABY'S LIFE.

FROM THE MOMENT OF CONCEPTION, YOU AND YOUR GROWING BABY GO THROUGH A MULTITUDE OF EXTRAORDINARY CHANGES. YOUR PREGNANCY IS DATED FROM THE FIRST DAY OF YOUR LAST PERIOD. THE AVERAGE LENGTH OF PREGNANCY IS 40 WEEKS AND IT IS DIVIDED INTO THREE PARTS, OR TRIMESTERS, WHICH LAST APPROXIMATELY THREE MONTHS EACH.

PREGNANCY AND CHILDBIRTH WILL CHALLENGE YOUR BODY MORE THAN ANYTHING YOU HAVE EXPERIENCED BEFORE.

BEING FULLY PREPARED IN MIND AS WELL AS IN BODY IS ALSO IMPORTANT TO MAINTAIN YOUR WELL-BEING.

THIS BOOK GIVES SPECIFIC ADVICE ABOUT A **BALANCED DIET**, WHICH SUPPLEMENTS TO TAKE, WHICH FOOD AND DRINKS TO AVOID, AND **HOW TO EXERCISE SAFELY** DURING PREGNANCY AND BEYOND.

FROM PRECONCEPTION TO BIRTH, WHAT YOU EAT AND DRINK CAN AFFECT YOUR PREGNANCY: HOW QUICKLY YOU CONCEIVE, YOUR HEALTH DURING PREGNANCY, YOUR EXPERIENCES OF PREGNANCY AND LABOR, AND THE HEALTH OF YOUR BABY—NOT ONLY WHILE HE IS GROWING INSIDE YOU, BUT ALSO LONG INTO HIS FUTURE.

Nutrition

J UST BECAUSE YOU ARE PREGNANT DOES NOT MEAN YOU GET TO EAT ANYTHING, AT ANY TIME YOU WANT. AS A PREGNANT WOMAN, THERE ARE A FEW RESTRICTIONS IN PLACE TO HELP KEEP YOU AND YOUR BABY SAFE AND HEALTHY. THERE WILL BE TIMES WHEN YOU WILL CRAVE FOR CERTAIN FOOD AND YOU WILL HAVE TO SHOW A LOT OF WILLPOWER.

THERE WILL ALSO BE MANY DIFFERENT TYPES OF FOOD THAT YOU SHOULD EAT BUT WILL NOT WANT TO DO SO BECAUSE THEY TASTE BLAND. WE WILL SHOW YOU HOW TO MANAGE SUCH FOOD AND MAKE THEM TASTE GREAT. IN FACT, THE INFORMATION IN THIS CHAPTER ALSO WILL HELP YOU MAKE A SHOPPING LIST THAT WILL MAKE IT ALMOST IMPOSSIBLE FOR YOU TO EAT THE WRONG TYPES OF FOOD. DURING PREGNANCY, THE KEY TO A HEALTHY BODY AND A HEALTHY CHILD IS EATING SIMPLE AND EATING RIGHT.

YOU NEED A LOT OF NUTRITION DURING PREGNANCY BECAUSE A LOT OF THE NUTRITION YOU ABSORB GOES TO YOUR CHILD. HOWEVER, THAT DOES NOT MEAN YOU EAT EVERYTHING IN SIGHT. ALTHOUGH YOU SHOULD

EAT MORE, RULES OF MODERATION AND VARIETY STILL APPLY.

NUTRITION ALREADY HOLDS A LOT OF VALUE TO WOMEN.

LIST OF HEALTHY & UNHEALTHY FOODS

OMEGA-3 RICH FISH

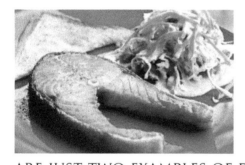

EATING FISH RICH IN OMEGA-3 FATTY ACIDS, ESPECIALLY DHA, IS A GREAT WAY TO IMPROVE THE DEVELOPMENT OF YOUR BABY'S BRAIN. SALMON AND LAKE TROUT ARE JUST TWO EXAMPLES OF FISH RICH IN OMEGA-3.

FURTHERMORE, WITH THE RIGHT AMOUNT OF OMEGA-3, NOT ONLY WILL YOUR CHILD SLEEP BETTER, YOU WILL EXPERIENCE LESS, IF ANY, POSTPARTUM DEPRESSION.

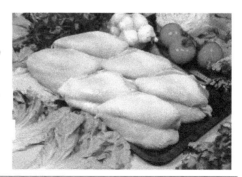

MEAT

MEAT IS VERY IMPORTANT FOR PREGNANT MOMS,

ESPECIALLY LEAN MEAT AS IT CONTAINS A LOW AMOUNT OF FAT AND A HIGH AMOUNT OF PROTEIN. THIS ESSENTIAL NUTRIENT IS REQUIRED TO HELP YOUR BABY'S BODY GROW. A PROTEIN DEFICIENCY COULD RESULT IN BIRTH DEFECTS.

HOWEVER, YOU MUST REMEMBER TO EAT LEAN MEAT AND STAY AWAY FROM ANY MEAT THAT HAS A HIGH AMOUNT OF FAT IN IT. IF YOU ARE A BACON LOVER, SAY GOODBYE TO IT.

MEAT IS ALSO HIGH IN IRON; AN ESSENTIAL COMPONENT OF BLOOD. WITHOUT AN ADEQUATE BLOOD SUPPLY, YOUR CHILD WILL NOT GET ENOUGH OXYGEN. THE DEVELOPMENT OF YOUR CHILD'S TEETH AND BONES WILL ALSO BE AFFECTED.

MEAT WILL ALSO:

- ❖ KEEP THE PLACENTA HEALTHY.
- ❖ YOUR BABY'S HORMONES IN CHECK.
- ❖ IMPROVE THE METABOLISM OF THE BABY.
- ❖ ENHANCE THE FORMATION OF BREAST MILK.

Vegetables

Vegetables are an important part of any pregnant woman's diet because they provide the body with a high amount of carbohydrate.

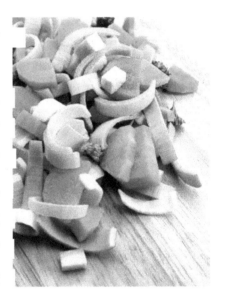

Carbohydrate is the number one nutrient that any pregnant woman requires. Carbohydrate is the single most important fuel source for the body. Without an ample supply of carbohydrate, your body will tire out faster.

Additionally, your child will not get its required amount of energy; resulting in poor growth. Vegetables also contain calcium, another essential vitamin during pregnancy.

However, moms-to-be need to remember that they require simple, not complex carbohydrates. Simple carbs are broken down much more

EFFICIENTLY BY THE BODY AND ARE THUS ESSENTIAL TO KEEPING OFF THE EXCESS BABY FAT.

MILK

MILK IS AN EXCEPTIONALLY IMPORTANT COMPONENT OF ANY PREGNANCY DIET BECAUSE MILK CONTAINS A HIGH AMOUNT OF CALCIUM, ESSENTIAL FOR PROPER STRUCTURAL GROWTH. CALCIUM IS ESSENTIAL FOR 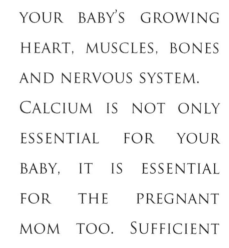 YOUR BABY'S GROWING HEART, MUSCLES, BONES AND NERVOUS SYSTEM. CALCIUM IS NOT ONLY ESSENTIAL FOR YOUR BABY, IT IS ESSENTIAL FOR THE PREGNANT MOM TOO. SUFFICIENT CALCIUM LEVELS REDUCE BLOOD PRESSURE AND BACK PAIN, NULLIFY MUSCLE CRAMPS, AND EVEN REDUCE THE PAIN EXPERIENCED DURING LABOR.

THIS IS ONE OF THE BIGGEST REASONS WHY MOMS-TO-BE ARE NOT ALLOWED TO SKIP BREAKFAST. A HEALTHY WHOLE GRAIN CEREAL WITH A FEW FRUITS, AND A

GLASS OF FRESHLY SQUEEZED JUICE, IS ONE OF THE BEST BREAKFAST IDEAS FOR ANY PREGNANT WOMEN.

FOODS TO AVOID

WHEN YOU ARE PREGNANT, THERE ARE MANY DIFFERENT FOODS YOU SHOULD AVOID. PREGNANCY IS NOT A LICENSE THAT ALLOWS YOU TO FEAST ON ANYTHING YOU WANT. HERE IS A LIST OF FOODS THAT YOU NEED TO AVOID AT ALL COSTS.

FAST FOOD

IF THERE IS ONE THING YOU NEED TO AVOID AT ALL COSTS DURING PREGNANCY, IT'S FAST FOOD. EVERYONE KNOWS FAST FOOD ISA GREASY, FAT-FILLED AND CHOLESTEROL PACKING MONSTROSITY.

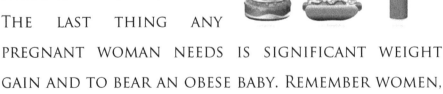

THE LAST THING ANY PREGNANT WOMAN NEEDS IS SIGNIFICANT WEIGHT GAIN AND TO BEAR AN OBESE BABY. REMEMBER WOMEN,

THE MORE FAT YOU EAT, THE HARDER THE TIME YOU WILL HAVE DURING LABOR.

Ready-to-eat

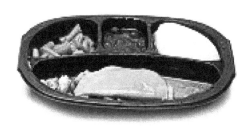

ANYTHING THAT IS READY TO EAT IS COMPLETELY OFF LIMITS TO PREGNANT WOMEN. YOU WILL BE DOING NOTHING BUT PACKING ON CALORIES; POSSIBLY THE ONLY THING SUCH FOOD IS GOOD FOR.

READY-TO-EAT MEALS AND SNACKS HAVE VERY LITTLE NUTRITIONAL CONTENT IN THEM AND SHOULD BE AVOIDED. ALL YOU WILL BE DOING IS GAINING WEIGHT. CONTRARY TO POPULAR BELIEF, EVEN READY-TO-EAT SALADS ARE OUT OF THE QUESTION. MANY CONTAIN A LOT OF ADDITIVES. FURTHERMORE, MANY CONTAIN FATTENING AND UNHEALTHY SALAD DRESSINGS. ALTHOUGH TASTY, YOU ARE BETTER OFF MAKING YOUR OWN SALAD. IT DOES NOT TAKE LONG AND IT IS DEFINITELY A LOT MORE NUTRITIOUS.

SOFT CHEESE

SOFT CHEESE AND PREGNANCY DO NOT GO WELL TOGETHER. THIS IS PRIMARILY BECAUSE SOFT CHEESE CAN CONTAIN LARGE AMOUNTS OF SATURATED FAT; A PREGNANT WOMAN'S WORST ENEMY. ALTHOUGH THIS IS NOT ALWAYS THE CASE, IT IS BETTER TO BE SAFE THAN SORRY.

ICE-CREAM

EVEN THOUGH THE PICTURE ON THE SIDE LOOKS ABSOLUTELY TEMPTING, THIS IS YET ANOTHER TYPE OF FOOD THAT YOU WILL HAVE TO STAY AWAY FROM.

THIS ONE IS PARTICULARLY FOR WOMEN WHO HAVE GESTATIONAL DIABETES. DURING PREGNANCY, THE LAST THING YOU NEED IS SUGARY 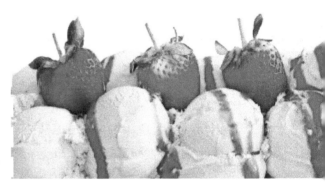 ICE-CREAM. ALL IT WILL DO IS PACK ON THE EXTRA POUNDS.

Making Shopping Lists

When most of us go shopping, we can hardly 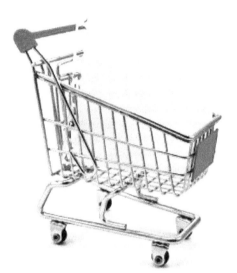 remember what we need to buy. We end up buying items we don't need because they were on sale. As a pregnant woman, you cannot afford to buy food that you don't need or should avoid.

If you are looking for a way to avoid unhealthy food and feast on healthy food, there is only one thing you can do; make a shopping list. Making a shopping list will ensure that you only buy what you need to buy and are not tempted to buy the big 2 liter soft ice-cream on sale.

To be honest, most of us can hardly remember what food we need to eat and which ones we need to avoid. We end up writing unhealthy food on our shopping list and this can be hazardous, for both you and your baby.

Therefore, if you want to ensure that you never put the wrong kind of food on your shopping list, have a friend (who has undergone pregnancy) check it for you. She will ensure that you have the right items on your list. In case you have put 'extra' items on your list, she will make sure they are off the list.

There are few experiences in your life that will demand as much of your body as pregnancy and childbirth.

Preparing yourself by eating as well as you can is hugely beneficial—a healthy body helps make your experience of conception, pregnancy, and labor a positive one.

Our diets have changed dramatically over the course of the last 50 years; it seems normal now to eat prepared, processed, and refined foods regularly rather than always making meals and

SNACKS FROM SCRATCH OURSELVES. HOWEVER, EATING ENOUGH OF THE RIGHT NUTRIENTS IS ONE OF THE MOST POSITIVE THINGS YOU CAN TAKE CONTROL OF. GOOD NUTRITION DOESN'T NEED TO BE ANY MORE COMPLICATED THAN THE GENERAL PRINCIPLES OF EATING A HEALTHY, BALANCED DIET—JUST BE AWARE THAT WHAT YOU STOCK IN YOUR CUPBOARDS AND FRIDGE AND PUT ON YOUR PLATE IS EVEN MORE IMPORTANT THAN USUAL, BOTH FOR YOUR FERTILITY AND ENERGY LEVELS AND FOR THE HEALTH OF YOUR DEVELOPING BABY. YOU DON'T HAVE TO FOLLOW A RIGID DIET OR EAT UNPLEASANT FOODS: IT'S ALL ABOUT EATING TWICE AS WELL (AND NOT TWICE AS MUCH) TO ENSURE YOU RECEIVE THE BEST NUTRIENTS FROM EVERY MOUTHFUL.

A BALANCED DIET ALLOWS YOUR BODY TO STORE ENOUGH OF THE RIGHT NUTRIENTS FOR A HEALTHY PREGNANCY AND FEEL IN PEAK CONDITION. EATING IN A CONSISTENT AND MEASURED WAY ALSO HELPS YOU TO KEEP YOUR WEIGHT WITHIN HEALTHY LIMITS, WHICH IS A FACTOR FOR SUCCESSFUL CONCEPTION. ONCE YOU BECOME PREGNANT, THE BENEFIT OF EATING A BALANCED DIET IS THAT YOU WILL BE SUPPLYING YOUR

BODY WITH THE BEST POSSIBLE DIET FOR FETAL GROWTH AND DEVELOPMENT AND PROVIDING YOURSELF WITH ENOUGH ENERGY TO DEAL WITH THE PREGNANCY.

AS SOON AS YOU CONCEIVE, YOU BECOME THE LIFELINE TO YOUR BABY—EVERYTHING YOU EAT, DRINK, AND BREATHE IS BROKEN DOWN INTO MOLECULES CONTAINING VALUABLE NUTRIENTS AND OXYGEN AND TRANSPORTED THROUGH YOUR BLOODSTREAM AND PLACENTA TO THE FETUS. SO IT'S IMPORTANT TO HAVE GOOD HABITS IN PLACE FROM THE START. THIS SECTION GIVES ADVICE ON HOW YOU CAN PREPARE FOR AND AID CONCEPTION, INCLUDING WHAT SUPPLEMENTS TO TAKE. ONCE YOU HAVE CONCEIVED, YOU CAN READ ABOUT EATING FOR ENERGY AND HEALTH, WHAT YOUR BABY NEEDS, THE BEST APPROACH IF YOU HAVE AN INTOLERANCE OR YOU FOLLOW A SPECIAL DIET FOR PERSONAL OR MEDICAL REASONS, WHICH FOODS TO AVOID, AND ADVICE ON SMOKING AND DRUGS.

AFTER THE BIRTH, YOU CAN LEARN ABOUT HOW TO BOOST YOUR RECOVERY THROUGH GOOD NUTRITION.

YOUR DIET CAN ADVERSELY AFFECT YOUR INTERNAL CHEMISTRY.

YOUR WEIGHT—WHETHER YOU'RE OVERWEIGHT OR UNDERWEIGHT—IS ALSO AN IMPORTANT FACTOR IF THERE ARE FERTILITY ISSUES, SINCE IT CAN DETERMINE WHETHER OR NOT YOU HAVE TOO LITTLE OR TOO MUCH ESTROGEN TO OVULATE. FOR A MAN, BEING UNDERWEIGHT CAN AFFECT THE QUALITY OF HIS SPERM. EAT THE RIGHT BALANCE OF HEALTHY, NUTRITIOUS.

IF YOU LEAD A HEALTHY LIFESTYLE AND EAT A GOOD, BALANCED DIET, YOU'VE ALREADY ESTABLISHED THE RIGHT PATTERN. IF NOT, MAKE POSITIVE CHANGES TO YOUR NUTRITION NOW TO HELP THE HEALTH OF YOUR SPERM AND EGGS (WHICH EACH TAKE THREE MONTHS TO DEVELOP) AND ESTABLISH THE NECESSARY RESERVES OF NUTRIENTS FOR A HEALTHY PREGNANCY. ALSO ELIMINATE, OR REDUCE TO WITHIN GUIDELINE LEVELS, ALCOHOL AND CAFFEINE, WHICH HAVE A DETRIMENTAL EFFECT ON CONCEPTION. EAT MORE PHYTOESTROGENS— FOUND IN LINSEED, WHOLE WHEAT, AND LENTILS—TO BALANCE HORMONES IN BOTH PARTNERS, AND EAT A COLORFUL RANGE OF

ANTIOXIDANT-RICH FOODS TO BOOST THE QUALITY AND MOTILITY OF SPERM.

EAT A VARIETY OF FOODS FROM EACH OF THESE GROUPS IN THE RIGHT PROPORTIONS FOR OPTIMUM NUTRITIONAL BENEFITS AT EVERY MEAL. THE BREAKDOWN OF THESE HEALTHY FOODS EQUATES TO APPROXIMATELY FIVE TO SIX PORTIONS OF FRESH VEGETABLES, TWO PORTIONS OF FRESH FRUIT, AND THREE PORTIONS EACH OF PROTEIN AND UNREFINED CARBOHYDRATES PER DAY.

FRESH FRUIT AND VEGETABLES

WHEN IT COMES TO FRUIT AND VEGETABLES, THE MORE COLORFUL THE BETTER. STRONG COLOR IS A SIGN THAT THEY ARE RICH IN VITAMINS AND MINERALS, AND HIGH IN PROTECTIVE ANTIOXIDANTS, WHICH HELP TO FIGHT FREE RADICALS IN THE BODY. EAT A WIDE COLOR RANGE OF VEGETABLES AND FRUIT FOR THE MAXIMUM BENEFITS.

FRUIT CONTAINS FRUCTOSE, A TYPE OF SUGAR, SO A COUPLE OF PORTIONS A DAY WILL GIVE YOU FIBER AND VITAMINS WITHOUT OVERLOADING ON SUGAR.

Choose fish, poultry, beans, and nuts.

Limit red meat and avoid bacon and processed meats. Steam, grill, or bake fish and meat.

Eat a variety of whole grains (such as whole-wheat bread, whole-grain pasta, and brown rice).
Limit or avoid refined grains (such as white rice and white bread).

Essential supplement

Whether you're already pregnant or trying to get pregnant, start taking folic acid as soon as you can.

Folic acid. is the synthesized version of vitamin B9. When it occurs naturally in food, it is known as folate and is present in leafy green vegetables such as cabbage. Studies show that our bodies are better at using the synthesized version so look for supplements that contain 5-methyltetrahydrofolic acid, which is already "biologically active."

IRON NEEDS. IT IS USUALLY BETTER TO GET YOUR IRON NEEDS FROM YOUR DIET. THIS IS BECAUSE IRON SUPPLEMENTS CAN HAVE THE SIDE EFFECT OF CAUSING CONSTIPATION, WHICH PREGNANT WOMEN ARE ALREADY SUSCEPTIBLE TO. EATING IRON-RICH, HIGH-FIBER FOODS IS GOOD FOR TACKLING BOTH CONSTIPATION AND LOW IRON LEVELS. INCLUDE MORE LEAN RED MEAT, GREEN LEAFY VEGETABLES, NUTS SUCH AS PEANUTS, AND DRIED FRUIT IN YOUR DIET. IT'S USUAL DURING PREGNANCY TO FEEL MORE TIRED THAN NORMAL, PARTICULARLY IN THE FIRST AND LAST TRIMESTERS. HOWEVER, IF YOU ARE EXTREMELY LETHARGIC, PALE, AND SUFFERING FROM HEART PALPITATIONS AND/OR SHORTNESS OF BREATH, YOU COULD BE ANEMIC. IF YOU ARE, YOUR DOCTOR WILL DISCUSS IRON SUPPLEMENTATION. IN ADDITION, CONSIDER CUTTING OUT CAFFEINE ENTIRELY SINCE THIS CAN HAMPER IRON ABSORPTION.

FOODS TO LIMIT OR AVOID

Although there is usually only a small risk that foods such as these may prove harmful to your baby, they are best avoided or limited while you are pregnant.

Banned foods Cured meats and unpasteurized cheeses should be avoided.

Cheese

Any unpasteurized cheese. Soft mold-ripened cheeses, such as Camembert and Brie. Uncooked soft blue cheeses, such as Roquefort.In rare cases, **CHEESE** may carry the listeria bacteria. Listeriosis (listeria infection) may cause only mild, flu-like symptoms in you, but it can be harmful to your baby and in severe cases can lead to brain damage.

YOU CAN EAT HARD CHEESES AND HARD
BLUE CHEESES (SUCH AS PARMESAN, GOUDA,
CHEDDAR AND STILTON). SOFT CHEESES
MADE WITH PASTEURIZED MILK, FOR
EXAMPLE COTTAGE CHEESE, CREAM CHEESE,
MOZZARELLA, FETA, AND RICOTTA.

MEAT RAW OR UNDERCOOKED RED MEAT. COLD
CUTS AND LUNCHEON MEATS. **UNDERCOOKED
MEAT** MAY BE INFECTED WITH THE OXOPLASMOSIS
PARASITE AND COLD CUTS MAY CONTAIN
LISTERIA. BOTH MAY HARM YOUR BABY. TOO
MUCH VITAMIN A CAN CAUSE BIRTH DEFECTS
AND HARM YOUR BABY'S LIVER.
YOU CAN EAT MEAT THAT HAS BEEN COOKED TO
A SAFE TEMPERATURE IS FINE TO EAT.

SEAFOOD

UNCOOKED SHELLFISH. AVOID SHARK, MARLIN,
AND SWORDFISH, WHICH CONTAIN HIGH LEVELS
OF MERCURY. HIGH LEVELS OF MERCURY, FOUND
IN CERTAIN FISH, CAN BE HARMFUL TO YOUR
BABY'S NERVOUS SYSTEM.

YOU CAN EAT OILY FISH, BUT ONLY ONCE OR TWICE A WEEK, SINCE IT MAY CONTAIN TOXINS SUCH AS PCBS AND DIOXINS (AS WELL AS LOTS OF GOOD NUTRIENTS).

EGGS RAW EGGS AND RAW EGG PRODUCTS SUCH AS MAYONNAISE AND MOUSSE. UNDERCOOKED EGGS. EAT ONLY IF THE YOLK AND WHITE ARE SOLID. THERE IS A TINY RISK THAT **RAW EGGS** MAY CONTAIN THE SALMONELLA BACTERIA.

YOU CAN EAT CHOOSE EGGS STAMPED TO SHOW THAT THEY HAVE BEEN LAID IN CONDITIONS FOLLOWING THE STRICTEST HYGIENE.

SUGAR SUBSTITUTES

MOST ARTIFICIAL SWEETENERS ARE CONSIDERED SAFE IN MODERATION DURING PREGNANCY, INCLUDING SUCRALOSE AND ASPARTAME.

ALCOHOL WE KNOW THAT ALCOHOL CROSSES THE PLACENTA, MEANING ANY ALCOHOL YOU DRINK CAN MAKE ITS WAY INTO YOUR BABY'S SYSTEM. BECAUSE THE LIVER **IS ONE OF THE LAST ORGANS TO** DEVELOP IN THE FETUS, YOUR BABY CAN'T DETOXIFY THE EFFECTS. THIS RAISES THE CONCENTRATION OF ALCOHOL IN THE BABY'S BLOOD AND STARVES THE BABY OF OXYGEN.

CAFFEINE THIS IS PRESENT IN MUCH MORE THAN JUST COFFEE AND TEA CHOCOLATE, CARBONATED DRINKS, AND ENERGY DRINKS, TO NAME A FEW. GUIDELINES ARE THAT, DURING PREGNANCY, WOMEN SHOULDN'T DRINK MORE THAN TWO CUPS OF INSTANT COFFEE A DAY.

Herbal teas contain no caffeine, but they aren't regulated by the Food and Drug Administration, and there's not much research about the effects of many herbs on pregnancy. Stick to decaffeinated black teas instead. If you want to drink fruit or ginger teas, read the ingredients carefully to make sure that no herbs are present.

Cigarettes and recreational drugs (such as cocaine and marijuana) are known to pose significant health risks to an unborn child, resulting in:

- Low birthweight brain or lung damage
- Miscarriage
- Babies born with "addiction"

First Trimester: A Diet to Get You Started

THIS CHAPTER PROVIDES CLEAR-CUT GUIDELINES ON WHICH FOODS TO AVOID, AND EXPLAINS HOW HEALTHY EATING CAN OPTIMIZE YOUR BABY'S EARLY DEVELOPMENT. SENSIBLE EXERCISE ADVICE AND RELAXATION TECHNIQUES HELP YOU DEAL WITH COMMON PREGNANCY CONCERNS, AND DEVELOP STAMINA AND FOCUS FOR LABOR.

ONCE A SPERM FERTILIZES AN EGG, YOUR BABY BEGINS LIFE. AFTER SEVERAL DAYS, IT BURROWS INTO THE LINING OF THE UTERUS.
THE PLACE WHERE IT IMPLANTS WILL DEVELOP INTO THE PLACENTA.

THE FIRST TRIMESTER IS VERY IMPORTANT FOR THE MOTHER AND THE BABY. FOR MOST WOMEN IT IS COMMON TO FIND OUT ABOUT THEIR PREGNANCY AFTER THEY HAVE MISSED THEIR MENSTRUAL CYCLE. SINCE, NOT ALL WOMEN NOTE THEIR MENSTRUAL CYCLE AND DATES OF INTERCOURSE, IT MAY CAUSE

SLIGHT CONFUSION ABOUT THE EXACT DATE OF CONCEPTION. THAT IS WHY MOST WOMEN FIND OUT THAT THEY ARE PREGNANT ONLY AFTER ONE MONTH OF PREGNANCY.

IT IS GENERALLY GOOD PRACTICE TO NOTE THE DATES THAT YOU HAVE HAD UNPROTECTED SEXUAL INTERCOURSE ON. THIS WILL GREATLY HELP THE DOCTOR IN CALCULATING THE DATE OF CONCEPTION AND THE DATE OF DELIVERY. PLUS, IT WILL HELP YOU CREATE A HEALTHY DIET PLAN FOR YOURSELF AND THE BABY.

EARLY PREGNANCY SYMPTOMS YOU MAY BE EXPERIENCING SYMPTOMS SUCH AS FOOD CRAVINGS, MORNING SICKNESS, EXTREME FATIGUE, AND MOOD SWINGS. THESE OFTEN FADE.

PRENATAL APPOINTMENTS YOUR FIRST APPOINTMENT TAKES PLACE AT AROUND 6 TO 8 WEEKS. IT WILL BE REALLY THOROUGH AND YOU'LL BE ABLE TO ASK THE DOCTOR ANY PREGNANCY-RELATED QUESTIONS THAT YOU MAY

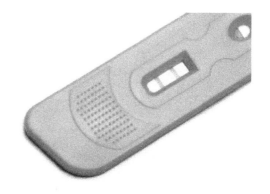

HAVE.

AS MENTIONED EARLIER THE FIRST TRIMESTER IS THE MOST IMPORTANT AND CRITICAL ONE IN EVERY PREGNANCY. A BABY DEVELOPS ITS VITAL ORGANS LIKE LUNGS, BRAIN AND HEART, IN THIS TRIMESTER. CARE TAKEN IN THIS TRIMESTER REALLY PAYS OFF DURING THE WHOLE PREGNANCY AND EVEN AFTER DELIVERY. YOU ARE ABLE TO HAVE A HEALTHY BABY AND KEEP YOUR BODY HEALTHY DURING THE WHOLE PREGNANCY AND POST-PREGNANCY PERIOD.

DAYS 1–14 THE COUNTDOWN OF YOUR PREGNANCY BEGINS WITH YOUR PERIOD—THE START OF THE FERTILITY CYCLE.

SINCE IT IS OFTEN HARD TO BE SURE OF THE EXACT DATE WHEN FERTILIZATION TAKES PLACE, THE FIRST DAY OF YOUR LAST MENSTRUAL PERIOD (LMP) IS USED AS A MARKER. IN THE FIRST TWO WEEKS THE BODY IS RESETTING THE FERTILITY CYCLE: IN THE FIRST WEEK THE PREVIOUS MONTH'S UTERINE LINING SHEDS; IN THE SECOND WEEK, THE UTERINE LINING HAS BEGUN TO THICKEN IN PREPARATION FOR THE NEXT OPPORTUNITY TO CONCEIVE A BABY.

2 WEEKS A MATURE EGG IS RELEASED FROM THE OVARIES AND IF A SPERM FERTILIZES IT, A BABY IS CONCEIVED.

THE ZYGOTE WILL SIGNAL ITS EXISTENCE TO THE PITUITARY GLAND IN YOUR BRAIN. A NEW HORMONE IS RELEASED CALLED HUMAN CHORIONIC GONADOTROPHIN (HCG) THAT OVERRIDES YOUR USUAL MONTHLY CYCLE.

3 WEEKS AMAZING THINGS ARE HAPPENING INSIDE YOUR BODY, AND SOME WOMEN MAY EXPERIENCE EARLY SIGNS.

HORMONES, INCLUDING ESTROGEN AND PROGESTERONE, SURGE THROUGH YOUR BODY TO HELP THE BLASTOCYST SETTLE SAFELY. IT'S POSSIBLE TO EXPERIENCE VERY EARLY SYMPTOMS SUCH AS SORE BREASTS AND FATIGUE. WHEN THE EGG IMPLANTS, IT CAN CAUSE SOME SLIGHT BLEEDING OR "SPOTTING," BUT THIS BLEEDING SHOULD BE LIGHT, BRIEF, AND NOT PAINFUL.

WHEN THE EGG IMPLANTS, IT CAN CAUSE SOME SLIGHT BLEEDING OR "SPOTTING," BUT THIS BLEEDING SHOULD BE LIGHT, BRIEF, AND NOT PAINFUL.

4 WEEKS IF YOU MISS A PERIOD THIS WEEK, IT COULD BE THE FIRST TIME YOU WONDER, "AM I PREGNANT?"

YOU MIGHT EXPERIENCE A VARIETY OF PREGNANCY SYMPTOMS INCLUDING MORNING SICKNESS. THE LEVELS OF HUMAN CHORIONIC GONADOTROPHIN (HCG) HORMONE THE FERTILIZED EGG IS PRODUCING ARE HIGH ENOUGH NOW THAT A PREGNANCY TEST WILL REGISTER POSITIVE.

5 WEEKS YOU WON'T BE LOOKING PREGNANT BUT AS YOUR BODY ADAPTS TO THE PREGNANCY, YOU MIGHT WELL BE FEELING IT.

COMMON FIRST TRIMESTER SYMPTOMS COULD BE IN FULL SWING NOW. MOST OF THE TIME THEY FADE AFTER 12 WEEKS. IF YOU ARE SUFFERING FROM MORNING SICKNESS TRY EATING PLAIN FOODS AND TAKING GINGER. IF YOU CAN'T KEEP ANYTHING DOWN, SPEAK TO YOUR DOCTOR.

6 WEEKS ALTHOUGH THERE IS NO VISIBLE BELLY BUMP, IT DOESN'T MEAN YOUR BODY ISN'T CHANGING IN OTHER WAYS.

YOUR METABOLISM SPEEDS UP, YOUR LUNGS ARE WORKING HARDER, AND YOUR BLOOD VOLUME IS ALREADY INCREASING. DON'T BE SURPRISED TO FIND A LITTLE WEIGHT GAIN ALREADY, EVEN THOUGH THERE'S NO SIGN OF A BELLY. YOUR BLOOD PRESSURE DROPS AS YOUR BLOOD VESSELS RELAX; THIS CAN CAUSE DIZZINESS SO TRY TO AVOID STANDING UP FOR LONG PERIODS. YOUR NIPPLES AND THE CIRCLES OF SKIN AROUND THEM (THE AREOLAE) MAY BE DARKER AND A MUCUS PLUG IN THE CERVIX SEALS OFF THE UTERUS TO PROTECT THE BABY FROM INFECTION.

7 WEEKS THOUGH YOU STILL CANNOT FEEL THE BABY INSIDE YOU, THE HEART CAN BE SEEN BEATING ON AN ULTRASOUND NOW.

YOUR UTERUS IS GRADUALLY EXPANDING, AND YOU MAY FIND THAT YOUR WAISTLINE IS THICKER. YOUR BREASTS WILL BE HEAVIER AND MAY FEEL TENDER AS THEY START TO ADAPT FOR BREAST-FEEDING. HORMONAL SURGES CAN ALSO BRING SKIN CHANGES, AND YOU MAY FIND YOU SUDDENLY GET ACNE, OR THAT YOUR SKIN DRIES OUT.

8 WEEKS As your body adapts to the hormonal changes of pregnancy, you may get sudden mood swings.

These first weeks are commonly marked by nausea, complete exhaustion, and mood swings. These are caused by hormonal and physiological changes that support your growing baby. Frequent trips to the bathroom are due to the increased production of urine by certain hormones and the growing uterus putting pressure on your bladder. Many women also have strange food cravings, or develop strong aversions to some foods.

9 WEEKS Your tiny baby is starting to move around, though you won't yet be able to feel this exciting action.

Your respiratory system adapts rapidly to help your body meet the demands of pregnancy. The ribs expand and the diaphragm moves up, enabling the lungs to take in more air, increasing oxygen absorption. You may feel the heat since the blood supply to the skin increases; to counter this, blood vessels dilate,

DISPERSING HEAT AND CONTROLLING YOUR BLOOD PRESSURE.

10 WEEKS THOUGH NOT OBVIOUS TO OTHERS, YOU MAY START TO NOTICE THAT YOUR BODY IS BEGINNING TO LOOK PREGNANT.

YOUR UTERUS STARTS TO MOVE UP AND OUT OF THE PELVIS AS IT GROWS. THIS SHIFT IN ITS POSITION MEANS LESS PRESSURE ON YOUR BLADDER. YOUR BREASTS CONTINUE TO GROW, AND YOU MAY GO UP TWO OR THREE BRA SIZES BY THE END OF THIS TRIMESTER. IT IS NORMAL TO FEEL INCREASINGLY BREATHLESS—YOUR BODY NEEDS TO TAKE IN MORE AIR, WHICH IS DIRECTED TOWARD THE BABY, UTERUS, AND PLACENTA—BUT MENTION IT TO YOUR DOCTOR IF YOU ARE ALARMED.

11 WEEKS YOU MAY SEE YOUR BABY FOR THE FIRST TIME ON YOUR FIRST ULTRASOUND.

YOU MAY NEED TO ADJUST YOUR WAISTBAND OR OPT FOR LOOSER-FITTING GARMENTS. PREGNANCY HORMONES CAN MEAN YOUR NIPPLES AND AREOLAE DARKEN AND BECOME BIGGER. BY NOW, UP TO A

QUARTER OF THE BLOOD PUMPED AROUND YOUR BODY IS BEING SENT TO THE UTERUS TO SUPPORT THE RAPID GROWTH OF YOUR BABY AND THE PLACENTA.

12 WEEKS WITH NAUSEA AND FATIGUE FADING AWAY, YOU ARE LIKELY TO FEEL MORE INVIGORATED.

SOME OF THE MORE UNPLEASANT SYMPTOMS OF EARLY PREGNANCY MAY START TO RECEDE, AND YOU MAY FEEL GREAT RELIEF AS YOUR APPETITE RETURNS, AND YOUR ENERGY LEVELS INCREASE. THE HORMONE HCG FALLS SIGNIFICANTLY NOW, WHICH MAY BE BEHIND THE NAUSEA SUBSIDING. FOR SOME WOMEN, NAUSEA CAN CONTINUE TO AROUND WEEK 20. IF THIS IS THE CASE, REST ASSURED THAT YOUR BABY WILL STILL BE GETTING ALL THE NUTRIENTS SHE NEEDS, EVEN IF YOU ARE SUFFERING!

DURING THE FIRST TRIMESTER YOU WILL GAIN SOME WEIGHT, BUT YOU DON'T REALLY NEED A LOT OF EXTRA CALORIES. JUST INCREASE THE DAILY INTAKE BY 200-300 CALORIES. YOU 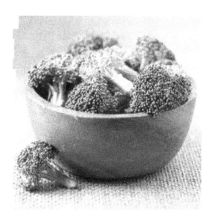 SHOULD BE EATING FOODS THAT ARE RICH IN FOLATES. FOLATE-RICH FOODS CONTAIN FOLIC ACID, WHICH ASSISTS IN THE BABY'S GROWTH. ASIDE, FROM EATING FOLATE-RICH FOODS, YOU SHOULD ALSO TAKE A DAILY SUPPLEMENT OF FOLIC ACID OF 400 MCG. FOLIC ACID HELPS WITH THE BABY'S PHYSICAL DEVELOPMENT.

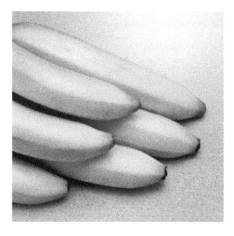

EXAMPLES OF FOLATE-RICH FOODS ARE BROCCOLI, ASPARAGUS, ORANGES, EGGS, BRAN FLAKES, ETC. ANOTHER NUTRIENT THAT IS IMPORTANT DURING THE FIRST TRIMESTER IS VITAMIN A. IT HELPS WITH

THE DEVELOPMENT OF THE BABY'S ORGANS AND RESPIRATORY, NERVOUS AND CIRCULATORY SYSTEMS. THIS NUTRIENT SHOULD BE TAKEN THROUGHOUT THE PREGNANCY.

THOUGH, THE FIRST TRIMESTER IS CRUCIAL FOR THE BABY'S GROWTH, THE MOTHER IS USUALLY FEELING TOO NAUSEOUS TO EAT ANYTHING. THEREFORE, SNACKING MAY BE A GOOD IDEA. VITAMIN B6 MAY BE HELPFUL IN THIS CASE TO EASE THE QUEASINESS OF MORNING SICKNESS. EXAMPLES OF VITAMIN B6-RICH FOODS ARE BANANAS, BLACK EYED BEANS, WHOLEGRAIN TOAST, SALMON, ETC.

Meal Plans

Making a meal plan helps you stay on the right track. Here are three meal plans, perfect for each month of the first trimester:

First Month

Meals / Days	Breakfast	Lunch	Dinner
Monday	1 glass of orange juice. A bowl of porridge made with milk. Flavored with 1 tbsp apple puree and pinch of cinnamon.	1 Banana. Smoked chicken with some avocado salad on the side.	Chicken cacciatore with brown rice.
Tuesday	1 glass fruit smoothie. Scotch pancakes	A bunch of grapes. Baked potato	Beef and black eye bean casserole.

	TOPPED WITH GREEK YOGURT, GINGER AND CHOPPED FRESH FRUIT.	WITH COTTAGE CHEESE.	
WEDNESDAY	1 GLASS OF CRANBERRY JUICE. A BOWL OF BRAN FLAKES WITH SEMI-SKIMMED MILK AND A SLICED BANANA.	1 APPLE. BROCCOLI AND PEA SOUP WITH A CRUSTY WHOLE-WHEAT ROLL.	SAUSAGE AND APPLE CASSEROLE
THURSDAY	1 CUP OF GREEN TEA. A BOWL OF PORRIDGE MADE WITH MILK. FLAVORED IT WITH 1 TBSP OF TINNED	A BOWL OF PAPAYA. FETA SALAD COUSCOUS.	CREAMY FISH PIE SALMON AND HADDOCK WITH ASPARAGUS.

BERRIES.

FRIDAY	WHOLEGRAIN TOAST SPREAD WITH PEANUT BUTTER	A SLICE OF MELON. SOFT CHEESE AND CRANBERRY WRAP WITH WATERCRESS.	LAMB CHOPS WITH POTATOES, PEAS AND BROCCOLI.
SATURDAY	A BOWL OF GREEK YOGHURT MIXED WITH 1 TBSP CHOPPED DRIED FRUIT AND MUESLI.	1 KIWI. WATERCRESS AND SALMON SALAD.	PASTA WITH LOW-FAT GARLIC BREAD.
SUNDAY	SCRAMBLED EGGS ON TOASTED BAGEL.	ROAST CHICKEN WITH POTATOES, CARROTS AND BROCCOLI. APPLE.	TOFU AND BUTTERNUT SQUASH FLAN.

Second Month

Meals / Days	Breakfast	Lunch	Dinner
Monday	1 glass of orange juice. A bowl of muesli with plain yoghurt and chopped apple.	1 banana. Smoked chicken with some avocado salad on the side.	Spanish chicken with couscous.
Tuesday	A yoghurt drink. A bowl of bran flakes with semi-skimmed milk and a sliced banana.	1 orange. Broccoli and pea soup.	Grilled pork chop with sweet potato mash, asparagus and green beans.
Wednesday	A fruit smoothie. 2 slices of	A bunch of grapes. Soft cheese	Brown rice chicken and

	WHOLEGRAIN TOAST WITH LOW-FAT SOFT CHEESE.	AND CRANBERRY WRAP WITH WATERCRESS.	MUSHROOM RISOTTO.
THURSDAY	A CUP OF GREEN TEA.		
	A BOWL OF GREEK YOGHURT MIXED WITH GINGER, CHOPPED MANGO AND 1 TBSP GRANOLA.	1 APPLE. MINESTRONE WITH A CRUSTY WHOLEGRAIN ROLL.	BAKED SALMON WITH POTATOES, SWEET CORN AND BROCCOLI.
FRIDAY		A SLICE OF MELON.	
	A FRUIT SMOOTHIE. 2 TOASTED CRUMPETS WITH PEANUT BUTTER.	BAKED POTATO WITH CHERRY TOMATOES AND COTTAGE CHEESE, CHOPPED CUCUMBER	BEEF AND BLACK BEAN CASSEROLE.

		AND SPRING ONIONS	
SATURDAY	1 GLASS OF APPLE JUICE. 2 RASHERS OF GRILLED BACON AND TOMATOES ON A SLICE OF WHOLEGRAIN TOAST.	CHOPPED MANGO AND PINEAPPLE. SARDINE MINCE ON WHOLEGRAIN TOAST WITH SLICED TOMATOES.	MACARONI AND CHEESE WITH SPINACH AND CHERRY TOMATOES.
SUNDAY	1 GLASS OF ORANGE JUICE. A BOWL OF PORRIDGE WITH 1 TSP OF HONEY AND 1 TBSP OF SULTANAS.	ROAST BEEF WITH ROASTED PARSNIPS AND CARROTS, WITH A PEAS AND ONION GRAVY. APPLE AND RASPBERRY FOOL.	A WELSH RAREBIT.

Third Month

MEALS	BREAKFAST	LUNCH	DINNER
DAYS			
MONDAY	1 GLASS OF CRANBERRY JUICE. TOASTED WHOLEGRAIN BAGEL WITH LOW-FAT SOFT CHEESE AND SLICED TOMATO.	1 ORANGE. EDAM AND PICKLE WHOLEGRAIN SANDWICH.	GRIDDLED CHICKEN BREAST WITH MANGO SALSA, NEW POTATOES AND PEAS
TUESDAY	A FRUIT SMOOTHIE. A BOWL OF WHOLEGRAIN CEREAL WITH SEMI-SKIMMED MILK AND 1 TBSP OF CHOPPED DRIED	1 APPLE. BAKED POTATO WITH SPRING ONIONS AND COTTAGE CHEESE.	CREAMY FISH PIE OF HADDOCK AND SALMON WITH PEAS.

	FRUITS.		
WEDNESDAY	1 GLASS OF APPLE JUICE GREEK YOGHURT WITH GINGER, WITH DRIED FRUIT AND NUTS AND 1 TBSP OF MUESLI.	1 PEAR. SMOKED CHICKEN AND AVOCADO SALAD WITH RYE CRACKERS.	PORK WITH ABAKED POTATO AND MUSHROOM, LOW-FAT CRÈME FRAICHE SAUCE.
THURSDAY	A FRUIT SMOOTHIE. 2 SLICES OF WHOLEGRAIN TOAST WITH 1 BOILED EGG	A SLICE OF MELON. PUMPKIN SOUP AND A CRUSTY ROLL.	BAKED SALMON WITH SWEET POTATO WEDGE SAND CORN ON THE COB.
FRIDAY	A YOGHURT DRINK. BRAN FLAKES WITH SEMI-SKIMMED	1 KIWI. EGG, WATERCRESS AND TOMATO BAGUETTE.	MOUSSAKA.

	MILK AND SLICED BANANA.		
SATURDAY		1 BANANA.	
	FRUIT SMOOTHIE AND A LOW-FAT BERRY MUFFIN	SOFT CHEESE AND CRANBERRY WRAP WITH WATERCRESS.	PENNE WITH TURKEY STRIPS, GREEN BEANS AND PEAS.
SUNDAY	1 GLASS OF ORANGE JUICE. TOASTED BAGEL WITH PEANUT BUTTER.	ROASTED PORK WITH GREEN BEANS. APPLE AND PEAR CRUMBLE.	TOFU AND BUTTERNUTSQUASH FLAN.

Second Trimester: A Diet for Those Cravings

AFTER THE FIRST TRIMESTER, OR WHEN YOU'VE HAD YOUR FIRST ULTRASOUND, IS A GOOD TIME TO TELL THE WIDER WORLD ABOUT YOUR PREGNANCY.

EXERCISE KEEP ACTIVE AND HEALTHY. YOUR REGULAR EXERCISE MAY BE TOO STRENUOUS NOW, SO ADAPT YOUR ROUTINE AND CONSIDER EXERCISE CLASSES ESPECIALLY TAILORED FOR PREGNANT WOMEN.

THE SECOND TRIMESTER OF PREGNANCY IS KNOWN AS THE MOST ENJOYABLE AND RELAXED PERIOD. IT IS OFTEN CALLED PREGNANCY'S 'HONEYMOON PHASE'! THE WORST IS OVER, THERE IS NO MORE NAUSEA AND YOU ARE STARTING TO GET USED TO BEING PREGNANT.

WHEN YOU ARE 8 TO 14 WEEKS PREGNANT, YOUR BABY WILL BE MEASURED FROM CROWN TO RUMP AND YOU'LL BE GIVEN AN ESTIMATED DELIVERY DATE. KEEP IN MIND, THOUGH, THAT THERE'S A FIVE-WEEK RANGE WHEN BIRTH COULD HAPPEN. YOU WILL BE OFFERED A

NUCHAL TRANSLUCENCY TEST IF YOU ARE 11 TO 14 WEEKS.

THIS TRIMESTER IS FULL OF PHYSICAL CHANGES FOR YOUR ENTIRE BODY. YOU WILL NOTICE YOUR BREASTS GETTING LARGER AND YOUR BELLY GROWING AS THE BABY MAKES ROOM IN YOUR UTERUS. YOU WILL NOTICE STRETCH MARKS AROUND YOUR BREASTS AND BELLY. IT IS COMMON TO HAVE OCCASIONAL LEG CRAMPS AND DIZZINESS. THIS IS JUST YOUR BODY ADJUSTING TO THE PREGNANCY.

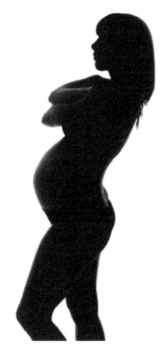

ALONG, WITH THESE BODY CHANGES THE CRAVING FOR FOOD ALSO GROWS. THIS IS BECAUSE THE BABY IS GROWING INSIDE OF YOU AND NEEDS NUTRITION. DURING THIS TRIMESTER YOU SHOULD NORMALLY GAIN 3 TO 4 POUNDS EVERY MONTH. GAINING WEIGHT IS SIGN OF A NORMAL PREGNANCY, SO DON'T BE AFRAID OF IT.

DURING THE LAST MONTH OF THIS TRIMESTER, YOU WILL EVEN START TO FEEL YOUR BABY MOVE. YOU MAY EVEN EXPERIENCE AN OCCASIONAL KICK OR JAB. FETAL

MOVEMENTS ARE SIGN OF A HEALTHY BABY AND ARE NECESSARY FOR THE BABY'S GROWTH AT THIS STAGE.

13 WEEKS CHANGES INSIDE YOUR BODY MEAN THAT YOU ARE GLOWING NOW. SIT BACK AND ENJOY THIS SETTLED PERIOD.

THE HORMONE RELAXIN IS SOFTENING YOUR JOINTS AND LIGAMENTS IN PREPARATION FOR BIRTH. THE DOWNSIDE IS THE ADDED STRAIN ON YOUR LIGAMENTS; YOU MAY START TO FEEL SOME DISCOMFORT. AS YOUR BLOOD VOLUME CONTINUES TO INCREASE, YOUR SKIN MAY START TO TAKE ON THE CHARACTERISTIC PREGNANCY "GLOW;" THIS, TOGETHER WITH YOUR MORE NOTICEABLE BELLY CAN START TO SIGNAL TO OTHERS THAT YOU'RE PREGNANT.

14 WEEKS YOUR PREGNANCY MAY BE BECOMING OBVIOUS, AND YOU MAY FEEL AN INCREDIBLE SENSE OF WELL-BEING.

IT'S NOT UNCOMMON TO HAVE A PERMANENTLY STUFFY NOSE, NOSEBLEEDS, AND SINUS HEADACHES. THESE ARE CAUSED BY THE EXTRA BLOOD FLOW TO THE MUCOUS MEMBRANES. NEW SYMPTOMS MAY EMERGE SUCH AS CONSTIPATION AND INDIGESTION. THESE ARE

THOUGHT TO BE SIDE EFFECTS OF THE HORMONES THAT MAKE YOUR DIGESTIVE SYSTEM SLUGGISH.

15 WEEKS IT IS NORMAL TO HAVE MIXED FEELINGS ABOUT YOUR CHANGING BODY SHAPE AND CURVES.

IN ADDITION TO GLOWING SKIN, YOU MAY ALSO FIND THAT YOUR HAIR IS FULLER AND MORE GLOSSY AS HORMONAL CONDITIONS PROLONG THE GROWTH PHASE OF HAIR AND LESS HAIR FALLS OUT ON A DAILY BASIS THAN USUAL. NAILS BECOME HEALTHIER AND STRONGER TOO.

16 WEEKS YOU WILL DEFINITELY START TO LOOK PREGNANT NOW, EVEN IF YOU DON'T FEEL THAT DIFFERENT.

A RISE IN THE PRODUCTION OF MELANIN, THE PIGMENT THAT GIVES YOUR SKIN AND HAIR ITS COLOR, CAN CREATE TEMPORARY SKIN CHANGES. DARK PATCHES, CALLED "CHLOASMA," MAY APPEAR ON YOUR CHEEKS, FOREHEAD, UPPER LIP, AND NECK. YOU MAY DEVELOP A DARK VERTICAL LINE DOWN YOUR ABDOMEN, CALLED A LINEA NIGRA. THESE LIGHTEN OR DISAPPEAR AFTER BIRTH

17 WEEKS THE BLOOM OF PREGNANCY MAY BE SHOWING IN YOUR SKIN, AND EVEN IN YOUR MOOD.

YOUR HEART IS NOW WORKING AT TWICE ITS NORMAL RATE TO PUMP THE INCREASED BLOOD VOLUME AROUND YOUR BODY. TO DEAL WITH THIS EXTRA VOLUME OF BLOOD AND STOP YOUR BLOOD PRESSURE FROM RISING, YOUR BLOOD VESSELS BECOME MORE FLEXIBLE AND DILATE. AS MORE BLOOD IS DIVERTED TO THE SKIN, YOU MAY LOOK POSITIVELY GLOWING AND HEALTHY. YOU MAY HAVE A RENEWED INTEREST IN SEX, HELPED BY THE INCREASED BLOOD FLOW TO THE PELVIC AREA.

18 WEEKS YOU MAY EXPERIENCE YOUR BABY'S EARLY, FLUTTERING MOVEMENTS. THESE ARE KNOWN AS "QUICKENING."

YOU MAY FEEL YOUR BABY MOVE FOR THE VERY FIRST TIME FROM THIS POINT. THESE EARLY MOVEMENTS ARE KNOWN AS "QUICKENING" AND CAN FEEL LIKE A FLUTTERY SENSATION. EACH WEEK YOUR UTERUS GROWS AROUND ⅜IN (1 CM), AND THE TOP OF THE UTERUS (THE FUNDUS) IS ALMOST LEVEL WITH YOUR

BELLY BUTTON. THE LIGAMENTS THAT SUPPORT THE PELVIC AREA STRETCH AND THIN, WHICH CAN CAUSE HIP AND BACK PAIN.

19 WEEKS YOU ARE ALMOST HALFWAY THROUGH YOUR JOURNEY. CONGRATULATIONS!

YOUR WEIGHT GAIN ACCELERATES IN THIS TRIMESTER. ON AVERAGE, WOMEN GAIN 1–2LB (0.5–1KG) PER WEEK FROM NOW UP UNTIL DELIVERY. YOUR BABY ACCOUNTS FOR ONLY SOME OF THIS EXTRA WEIGHT; THE REST IS INCREASED BLOOD VOLUME, BREAST SIZE, AMNIOTIC FLUID, AND FAT RESERVES. AS YOUR UTERUS CONTINUES TO MOVE UPWARD, PRESSING INTO THE STOMACH, AND PROGESTERONE RELAXES THE ABDOMINAL MUSCLES, DIGESTION CAN BECOME SLUGGISH.

YOU MAY SUFFER FROM HEARTBURN, INDIGESTION, AND CONSTIPATION, OR EXISTING SYMPTOMS MAY WORSEN.

20 WEEKS YOUR ULTRASOUND GIVES YOU A GLIMPSE OF YOUR WELL-FORMED BABY.

YOUR BELLY IS INCREASINGLY ROUNDED; IT SITS JUST BELOW YOUR BELLY BUTTON. YOUR EXTRA BLOOD

VOLUME HELPS SUPPLY THE ORGANS, WHICH ARE WORKING HARDER NOW TO SUPPORT YOU AND YOUR BABY.

21 WEEKS YOU ARE BECOMING MORE AWARE OF YOUR LIVELY BABY.

A LARGE PROPORTION OF YOUR INCREASED BLOOD VOLUME IS SENT TO YOUR UTERUS, AND THIS CHANGE IN THE DISTRIBUTION OF YOUR BLOOD CAN MAKE YOU FEEL DIZZY AT TIMES. YOUR BABY'S MOVEMENTS BECOME MORE OBVIOUS. ONCE YOU BECOME AWARE OF YOUR BABY'S PATTERN OF MOVEMENT (RATHER THAN THE ACTUAL NUMBER OF MOVEMENTS), THIS BECOMES A GOOD INDICATOR OF FETAL WELL-BEING. IF YOU DON'T FEEL ANY MOVEMENT FOR 24 HOURS, CONTACT YOUR DOCTOR.

22 WEEKS YOU MAY SEE SOME UNWANTED, THOUGH USUALLY TEMPORARY, SIDE EFFECTS.

AS THE UTERUS EXPANDS, THINNING THE SKIN'S COLLAGEN AND ELASTIN FIBERS, STRETCH MARKS MAY APPEAR. THESE FADE FROM RED OR DARK PURPLE TO A SHINY, PALER COLOR AFTER PREGNANCY. YOUR SKIN

MAY FEEL VERY DRY AND ITCHY. KEEPING HYDRATED AND USING AN UNPERFUMED MOISTURIZER CAN HELP. PAINFUL LEG-MUSCLE CRAMPS ARE A COMMON SYMPTOM DURING THIS TIME, WITH SPASMS OFTEN OCCURRING AT NIGHT. FLEXING THE FOOT AND MASSAGE CAN RELIEVE CRAMPS.

23 WEEKS KEEPING ACTIVE MEANS YOU WILL BE WELL PREPARED FOR THE BIRTH, AND PRIMED FOR A RAPID RECOVERY.

REGULAR GENTLE EXERCISE WILL HELP TO KEEP YOUR MUSCLES AND LIGAMENTS STRONG AND SUPPLE. THIS WILL ALSO HELP TO RELIEVE PREGNANCY COMPLAINTS SUCH AS BACKACHES. THERE'S ALSO SOME EVIDENCE THAT WOMEN WHO EXERCISE HAVE A SHORTER LABOR, AND THAT THE FETAL HEARTBEAT IS STRONGER. KEGEL EXERCISES ARE VERY IMPORTANT TOO, HELPING TO STRENGTHEN THE HAMMOCK OF MUSCLES THAT SUPPORT THE PELVIC AREA AND ORGANS, INCLUDING THE UTERUS.

24 WEEKS YOUR BABY MIGHT BE ACTIVE WHEN YOU WANT TO SLEEP—KICKING, YAWNING, AND EVEN HICCUPPING.

YOU WILL NOTICE YOUR ABDOMEN EXPANDING QUICKLY AS IT STRETCHES TO ACCOMMODATE YOUR RAPIDLY GROWING BABY. AS YOUR BELLY PROTRUDES OUTWARD AND RISES, IT PRESSES ON YOUR DIAPHRAGM, AND YOU MAY FEEL BREATHLESS. IT ALSO NUDGES AGAINST YOUR STOMACH, WHICH CAN LEAD TO HEARTBURN AND ACID REFLUX.

25 WEEKS AT THE CLOSE OF THE SECOND TRIMESTER, YOUR THOUGHTS MIGHT TURN TO THE BIRTH.

YOUR UTERUS CONTINUES TO MOVE UPWARD. YOUR ORGANS ARE COMPRESSED BY THE EXPANDING UTERUS, AND YOU COULD FEEL A BIT CRAMPED INSIDE. BLOOD VOLUME HAS INCREASED TO AROUND 8¾ PINTS (5LITERS), AND YOUR HEART IS WORKING HARD TO PUMP IT AROUND. THE BLOOD VESSELS HAVE RELAXED AS MUCH AS POSSIBLE, SO YOUR BLOOD PRESSURE MAY RISE A LITTLE NOW. IT IS NORMAL FOR YOUR HANDS, FEET, AND ANKLES TO SWELL AS A RESULT OF FLUID RETENTION (EDEMA).

SEVERE SWELLING WILL NEED TO BE MONITORED.

THE SECOND TRIMESTER IS THE EASIEST FOR THE MOTHER. NAUSEA AND MORNING SICKNESS HAVE PASSED AND YOU WILL FEEL A LOT MORE RELAXED AND 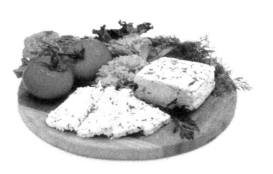 ENERGIZED. GAINING WEIGHT IS AN IMPORTANT PART OF THIS TRIMESTER.

DURING THIS TRIMESTER CALCIUM AND VITAMIN D ARE VERY IMPORTANT FOR THE MOTHER'S BODY. THESE WILL HELP YOUR BABY TO GROW STRONG BONES. EXAMPLES OF CALCIUM RICH FOODS ARE MILK, ALMONDS, YOGHURT, RICE AND CHEESE. EXAMPLES OF 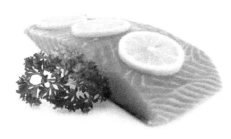 VITAMIN D RICH FOODS ARE FISH, EGG YOLK, SOY AND ORANGE JUICE.

OMEGA 3 FATTY ACIDS ALSO NEED TO BE AN IMPORTANT PART OF YOUR DIET. THEY HELP IN THE DEVELOPMENT OF THE BABY'S BRAIN. FISHES LIKE

SALMON AND MACKEREL ARE AN EXCELLENT SOURCE OF OMEGA 3 FATTY ACIDS.

IRON-RICH FOODS ARE IMPORTANT THROUGHOUT THE ENTIRE PREGNANCY. IRON WILL HELP YOUR BODY PRODUCE RED BLOOD CELLS WHICH ARE IMPORTANT FOR THE GROWING BABY. DRIED FRUITS, PORRIDGE, CHICKEN, LAMB, SPINACH AND GREEN VEGETABLES ARE A GOOD SOURCE OF IRON.

TO AVOID GAINING MORE WEIGHT THAN IS REQUIRED, YOU SHOULD FOLLOW A GOOD DIET PLAN. THIS WILL HELP YOU GAIN THE RIGHT AMOUNT OF WEIGHT REQUIRED FOR THE GROWTH OF THE BABY. GAINING TOO MUCH WEIGHT IS NOT A HEALTHY SIGN EITHER.

A MEAL PLAN IS THE BEST WAY TO KEEP YOUR PREGNANCY DIET RIGHT ON TRACK AND RECEIVE ALL THE NUTRITION REQUIRED FOR THE BABY IN THIS TRIMESTER. HERE ARE THREE MEAL PLANS, PERFECT FOR EACH MONTH OF THE SECOND TRIMESTER:

Fourth Month

MEALS / DAYS	BREAKFAST	LUNCH	DINNER
MONDAY	1 GLASS OF APPLE JUICE. PORRIDGE MADE IN MILK WITH 1 TBSP OF SULTANAS AND ALMONDS.	1 ORANGE. CIABATTA BREAD WITH HALLOUMI, SUNDRIED TOMATOES AND BASIL.	CHICKEN STIR FRY WITH NOODLES.
TUESDAY	1 GLASS OF PAPAYA SMOOTHIE. WHOLEGRAIN	1 PEAR. BROCCOLI AND PEA SOUP	CREAMY FISH PIE OF HADDOCK AND

	TOAST WITH SLICED BANANA AND PEANUT BUTTER.	CRUSTY WHOLEGRAIN ROLL.	SALMON WITH BROCCOLI.
WEDNESDAY	1 GLASS OF ORANGE JUICE. GREEK YOGHURT WITH WHEAT CEREALAND MIXED BERRIES.	A BOWL OF CHOPPED PAPAYA. 1 BAKED POTATO WITH COLESLAW AND TUNA.	MUSHROOM AND CELERY BAKED PASTA.
THURSDAY	A CUP OF HERBAL TEA. FROMAGE FRAIS (WHITE CHEESE) MIXED WITH 1 TBSP BERRY COMPOTE. TOASTED BAGEL WITH PEANUT BUTTER	1 KIWI. SMOKED CHICKEN AND AVOCADO SALAD.	PAN-FRIED TUNA STEAK. SWEET POTATO WEDGES AND SNAP PEAS ON THE SIDE.
FRIDAY	1 GLASS OF YOGHURT DRINK.PORRIDG	1 APPLE. HAM AND CHEESE	SWEET APPLE LAMB WITH COUSCOUS

	E MADE IN MILK WITH SLICED BANANAS.	WHOLEGRAIN SANDWICH.	AND SPINACH.
SATURDAY	SCRAMBLED EGGS WITH TOAST AND SPREAD ORANGE JUICE	TOASTED BAGEL WITH SMOOTH PEANUT BUTTER AND MASHED BANANA	VEGETABLE CURRY WITH MUSHROOM RICE.
SUNDAY	1 GLASS OF YOGHURT DRINK. SCOTCH PANCAKES WITH BLUEBERRIES.	ROAST PORK WITH ROAST PARSNIPS, SPRING GREENS AND POTATOES. RHUBARB CRUMBLE AND CUSTARD.	WATERCRESS AND CELERY SOUP WITH 1 WHOLEGRAIN ROLL.

Fifth Month

Meals / Days	Breakfast	Lunch	Dinner
Monday	1 glass of apple juice. Porridge made in milk with 1 tbsp of apple puree and a pinch of cinnamon.	1 apple. Pizza muffins.	Chicken cassoulet with spinach.
Tuesday	1 papaya smoothie a large bowl of fromage frais mixed with your choice of fresh fruits chopped and 1 tbsp	A few tinned peaches in juice. Baked potato with pineapple and cottage cheese.	Salmon with sweet potatowedges, sweetcorn and pine nuts.

	OF ALMONDS. SERVED WITH SCOTCH PANCAKES.		
WEDNESDAY	1 GLASS OF APPLE JUICE. WHEAT CEREAL WITH MILK AND SLICED BANANAS.	1 ORANGE. SALAD OF GRAPEFRUIT, AVOCADO, POMEGRANATE, SALAD LEAVES, WALNUTS AND FETA CHEESE.	PORK AND APPLE MEATBALLS SERVED WITH MASHED POTATOES AND MANGE TOUTS.
THURSDAY	1 CUP OF HERBAL TEA. PORRIDGE MADE IN MILK WITH 1 TBSP OF BERRY COMPOTE.	1 KIWI. BAKED POTATO AND BEANS.	GRILLED PLAICE FISH WITH WATERCRESS AND LOW-FAT OVEN CHIPS.
FRIDAY	1 GLASS OF	1 PEAR.	BEEF AND

	ORANGE JUICE. WHOLEGRAIN TOAST WITH SMOOTH PEANUT BUTTER.	SMOKED CHICKEN AND AVOCADO SALAD.	BLACK BEAN CASSEROLE.
SATURDAY	1 CUP OF HERBAL TEA. A LARGE BOWL OF GREEK YOGHURT WITH CHOPPED DRIED FRUITS OF YOUR CHOICE, ALMONDS AND 1 TBSP MUESLI.	HEALTHY BLT WITH GRILLED LEAN BACON, LETTUCE, THICK SLICES OF BEEF AND TOMATO ON GRANARY BREAD.	SPAGHETTI WITH SARDINES, TOPPED WITH ORANGES.
SUNDAY	1 YOGHURT DRINK.	ROAST CHICKEN	TORTILLA WITH SPICY TOMATO

SCRAMBLED EGGS SERVED ON TOASTED BAGEL.	WITH BROCCOLI, POTATOES AND CARROTS. BAKED APPLE WITH CUSTARD.	SAUCE, HAM, SPRING ONIONSAND CHEESE.

SIXTH MONTH

MEALS / DAYS	BREAKFAST	LUNCH	DINNER
MONDAY	1 GLASS OF APPLE JUICE. PORRIDGE MADE IN MILK WITH 1 TBSP OF SULTANAS AND ALMONDS.	1 PEAR. BAKED POTATO WITH CHEESY BAKED BEANS PEAR	CHICKEN KORMA (SPICY INDIAN CHICKEN CURRY) WITH STEAMED RICE.
TUESDAY	1 PAPAYA SMOOTHIE WHOLEGRAIN TOAST	1 ORANGE. CHEDDAR CHEESE AND TOMATO IN A	PAN-FRIED SALMON WITH PINE NUTS,

	WITH SLICED BANANAS.	WHOLEGRAIN ROLL	POTATOES AND WATERCRESS.
WEDNESDAY	1 GLASS OF ORANGE JUICE. WHEAT CEREAL WITH MIXED BERRY COMPOTE AND GREEK YOGHURT.	A SMALL BUNCH OF GRAPES CIABATTA BREAD WITH HALLOUMI CHEESE, BASIL AND SUNDRIED TOMATOES.	SWEET APPLE LAMB WITH MASHED POTATOES AND BROCCOLI.
THURSDAY	1 CUP OF HERBAL TEA. FROMAGE FRAIS WITH 1 TBSP OF BERRY COMPOTE. TOASTED BAGEL WITH PEANUT BUTTER.	1 APPLE. A BOWL OF CHOPPED PAPAYA. SALAD OF GRAPEFRUIT, AVOCADO, POMEGRANATE, SALAD LEAVES, WALNUTS AND FETA CHEESE.	SMOKED MACKEREL AND MUSHROOM FISHCAKES, SERVED WITH SPINACH AND CHERRY TOMATO SALAD.

FRIDAY	1 YOGHURT DRINK. PORRIDGE MADE IN MILK WITH SLICED BANANA.	1 KIWI. SMOKED SALMON, SOFT CHEESE ON BAGEL.	CHILLI CON CARNE SERVED WITH RICE.
SATURDAY	1 GLASS OF ORANGE JUICE. SCRAMBLED EGGS SERVED ON TOASTED BAGEL	1 BOWL OF CHOPPED PAPAYA. MUSHROOM AND CELERY BAKED PASTA.	HOMEMADE BURGERS WITH SALAD AND FRUITY COLESLAW.
SUNDAY	1 YOGHURT DRINK. SCOTCH PANCAKES WITH BLUEBERRIES.	FRUIT SALAD. ROAST BEEF, POTATOES, CAULIFLOWER AND CARROTS WITH CHEESE.	WATERCRESS AND CELERY SOUP WITH WHOLEGRAIN ROLL.

Third Trimester: A Diet to Keep Your Energy High

The third trimester is the most emotionally and physically challenging part of a pregnancy. The position and size of your baby may make is difficult for you to feel comfortable in any position. To top that, there is the anxiety of the approaching delivery date.

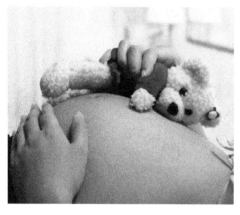

During this trimester you will experience continued growth of your breast, backaches, swelling of your feet and legs, and heartburn. As the delivery comes close you will also experience Braxton Hicks contractions. These are not real contraction, but rather a warm-up for the real thing.

Through all of this, your emotions will most likely be high as the anticipation and fear of childbirth grows inside of you. You may want to start spending time talking to your baby and

PLAN AHEAD FOR THE DUE DATE. DIVERT YOUR THOUGHTS INTO THE PLANNING PROCESS OF CHOOSING A HEALTHCARE PROVIDER FOR YOUR BABY AND A HOSPITAL FOR YOUR CHILD'S BIRTH.

26 WEEKS IT'S THE HOME STRETCH. YOUR BELLY IS A SOURCE OF PRIDE, AND YOU WILL MARVEL AS IT GROWS. DON'T BE SURPRISED IF YOUR BREASTS START LEAKING A LITTLE FLUID NOW. THIS PREMILK, CALLED COLOSTRUM, IS PRODUCED IN PREGNANCY, READY FOR YOUR BABY RIGHT AFTER BIRTH. YOU MAY FEEL A SENSE OF RELIEF AS YOUR REACH THE THIRD TRIMESTER.

27 WEEKS REASSURINGLY, BABIES WHO ARE BORN AT THIS STAGE IN PREGNANCY HAVE A 90-PERCENT SURVIVAL RATE.

WITH THE PRODUCTION OF AMNIOTIC FLUID SLOWING AND YOUR BABY BECOMING INCREASINGLY ACTIVE, YOU'RE LIKELY TO FEEL PLENTY OF KICKS. NOTE YOUR BABY'S PATTERN OF ACTIVITIES; IF THERE ARE CHANGES IN HIS NORMAL BEHAVIOR (SUCH AS SLOWING DOWN OR STOPPING COMPLETELY), YOU SHOULD REPORT THEM TO YOUR DOCTOR. SOME WOMEN DEVELOP A PREGNANCY "WADDLE" AS THEY GROW, CAUSED BY THEIR CHANGING SHAPE AND THE LOOSENING OF

LIGAMENTS AND TISSUES. THIS MIGHT BECOME MORE EXAGGERATED OVER THE COMING WEEKS. MANY WOMEN FIND THEY BECOME CLUMSIER AT THIS STAGE. BE CAREFUL ON SLIPPERY SURFACES SUCH AS THE SHOWER OR BATHTUB.

28 WEEKS AT THIS POINT, YOU MAY NOT REMEMBER HOW YOU FELT WITHOUT A BELLY.

YOUR BREASTS ARE GEARING UP FOR FEEDING YOUR BABY. PREGNANCY HORMONES INCREASE THE BLOOD FLOW TO THE BREASTS AND CAUSE CHANGES TO THE TISSUE, THE VEINS BECOME MORE PROMINENT, AND THEY MAY INCREASE IN SIZE. THE NIPPLE AREA, OR AREOLA, ALSO CONTINUES TO GROW AND DARKEN. YOU MAY NOTICE SMALL BUMPS KNOWN AS MONTGOMERY'S TUBERCULES FORMING AROUND YOUR NIPPLES.

29 WEEKS YOU MAY START TO FEEL SHARP KICKS FROM YOUR BABY.

YOUR LUNG CAPACITY HAS INCREASED AND YOUR RIBS HAVE SPREAD OUT SIDEWAYS TO HELP YOUR LUNGS WORK HARDER. THERE IS PRESSURE ON YOUR OTHER ORGANS; YOU MAY FIND SYMPTOMS SUCH AS

HEARTBURN, CONSTIPATION, AND PALPITATIONS WORSEN, AND YOU EXPERIENCE TWINGES, ACHES, AND PAINS.

30 WEEKS REVIEW YOUR BIRTH PLAN AROUND NOW. IT'S NOT TOO LATE TO MAKE CHANGES.

ALTHOUGH LABOR IS A COUPLE OF MONTHS OFF, YOUR UTERUS IS PREPARING FOR THE EVENT BY MAKING PRACTICE "BRAXTON HICKS" CONTRACTIONS—YOU MAY START TO NOTICE TIGHTENING SENSATIONS AROUND YOUR ABDOMEN AROUND NOW OR IN LATER WEEKS. THESE RANGE FROM BEING MILD TO A STRONGER CRAMP LIKE FEELING, BUT THEIR IRREGULARITY AND THE FACT THEY AREN'T VERY PAINFUL MEANS THIS ISN'T THE REAL THING.

31 WEEKS YOUR BABY MAY BE LYING IN ANY NUMBER OF POSITIONS.

YOUR BLOOD VOLUME PEAKS AROUND THIS TIME. THIS EXTRA VOLUME IS LARGELY DUE TO AN INCREASE IN THE PLASMA AND FLUID CONTENT OF THE BLOOD, WHILE THE NUMBER OF RED BLOOD CELLS REMAINS THE SAME. THIS MEANS THE RED BLOOD CELLS BECOME

LESS CONCENTRATED, A COMMON CAUSE OF ANEMIA IN LATE PREGNANCY. THERE'S NO NEED TO WORRY ABOUT THE BABY, THOUGH, SINCE HE WILL STILL RECEIVE ALL THE NUTRIENTS AND OXYGEN HE NEEDS TO THRIVE.

32 WEEKS NOW IS A GOOD TIME TO START THINKING ABOUT PRACTICAL PREPARATIONS.

THE SIZE OF YOUR BELLY PUTS PRESSURE ON YOUR VEINS; THIS CAN LEAD TO VARICOSE VEINS. GENTLE EXERCISE, REST, AND SUPPORT HOSE CAN BRING RELIEF, AND SYMPTOMS SHOULD SETTLE DOWN AFTER THE BIRTH. YOUR BELLY BUTTON MAY POP OUT AROUND NOW. IF THIS BOTHERS YOU, REST ASSURED THAT IT SHOULD GO BACK AFTER THE BIRTH.

33 WEEKS EACH DAY, YOUR BABY IS PREPARING FOR SURVIVAL IN THE OUTSIDE WORLD.

YOUR HEART WORKS EXTRA HARD NOW AS YOU APPROACH THE HOME STRETCH— YOUR HEART RATE INCREASES BY 10 TO 15 BEATS A MINUTE AND THE HEART WORKS UP TO 50 PERCENT HARDER. IT'S NOT UNCOMMON TO EXPERIENCE FLUTTERY PALPITATIONS; THESE ARE USUALLY HARMLESS, THOUGH MENTION

THEM TO YOUR DOCTOR IF ACCOMPANIED BY BREATHLESSNESS OR CHEST PAIN.

34 WEEKS PRACTICING RELAXATION TECHNIQUES WILL HELP YOU PREPARE FOR LABOR.

YOUR BABY IS MOST LIKELY TO BE LYING VERTICALLY BY THIS STAGE OF PREGNANCY, THOUGH OCCASIONALLY, BABIES ARE IN A DIAGONAL OR HORIZONTAL POSITION. AS YOUR BABY GETS BIGGER, HER MOVEMENTS ARE LIKELY TO FEEL STRONGER, MORE FREQUENT, AND HAVE A RECOGNIZABLE PATTERN NOW RATHER THAN SEEMING LIKE ISOLATED KICKS.

35 WEEKS YOUR BODY IS WELL AND TRULY GEARING UP FOR THE BIG DAY.

WITH LABOR APPROACHING, YOUR BABY'S HEAD MAY BEGIN TO "ENGAGE" (DESCEND INTO YOUR PELVIS), AND YOUR BELLY MAY SIT LOWER. THE RELEASE OF PRESSURE ON THE DIAPHRAGM MAKES IT EASIER TO BREATHE. THIS IS KNOWN AS "LIGHTENING." THE BABY'S HEAD NOW PRESSES ON YOUR BLADDER, WHICH MEANS FREQUENT BATHROOM STOPS AND INTERRUPTED SLEEP.

ACHES AND PAINS IN THE PELVIC AREA MAY WELL INCREASE

36 WEEKS MAKE SURE YOU HAVE A PLAN READY FOR WHEN YOU GO INTO LABOR.

BRAXTON HICKS CONTRACTIONS MAY BE OCCURRING WITH INCREASING REGULARITY, AND PRODUCTION OF THE HORMONE RELAXIN INCREASES, HELPING TO RELAX THE PELVIC LIGAMENTS AND TO SOFTEN THE CERVIX. A COMBINATION OF HORMONAL SURGES, ANXIETY ABOUT LABOR, LACK OF SLEEP, AND ACHES AND PAINS MAY LEAVE YOU FEELING A LITTLE VULNERABLE. MOOD SWINGS ARE QUITE COMMON IN THESE FINAL WEEKS.

37 WEEKS AT THIS POINT YOU ARE PROBABLY AS BIG AS YOU ARE GOING TO GET.

YOUR MOVEMENT MAY SLOW SINCE YOUR SIZE MAKES IT DIFFICULT TO MOVE QUICKLY AND MAINTAIN BALANCE. YOUR BREASTS ARE READY TO FEED YOUR BABY AT BIRTH. THE MILK DUCTS HAVE BRANCHED OFF, CREATING A TRANSPORTATION SYSTEM TO DELIVER MILK TO YOUR BABY.

38 WEEKS Double-check your birth plan; it's not too late to make changes.

You may feel very fatigued in these final stages since you carry all the extra weight of the fetus, uterus, and extra fluid. Your heart is working at full capacity. Taking some time to lie down increases the blood flow to your baby, and helps you rest and recuperate.

39 WEEKS Make sure you are clear on how to recognize the signs of labor.

It's best to take it easy now and conserve your energy for labor.

Combine rests with periods of gentle activity. You are likely to feel a mounting pressure in your pubic region and your baby may be partially or fully engaged in your pelvis, although in second and subsequent pregnancies, this often happens later on.

40 WEEKS Very soon you will be holding your new baby in your arms.

APPROXIMATELY 45 PERCENT OF WOMEN HAVEN'T GIVEN BIRTH AT 40 WEEKS. HOWEVER, THE MAJORITY DELIVER DURING THE NEXT WEEK AND ONLY 15 PERCENT GO ABOVE 41 WEEKS. YOU MIGHT BE OFFERED A "SWEEP" TO INDUCE LABOR.

LIST OF FOODS

THE THIRD TRIMESTER IS ONCE AGAIN A LITTLE TOUGH FOR THE EXPECTING MOTHER. THIS IS THE FINAL STRETCH AND SOON YOU WILL BE ABLE TO HOLD THE BABY IN YOUR HANDS. MOST IMPORTANT 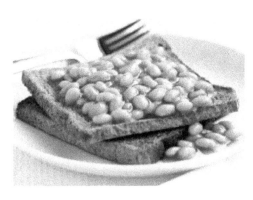 THROUGHOUT THE PREGNANCY PERIOD IS TO MAINTAIN A HEALTHY DIET. IT BENEFITS YOU AND THE GROWTH OF YOUR BABY. IN THIS TRIMESTER YOU CAN EXPECT TO GAIN AT LEAST A POUND EVERY WEEK. THE BABY WILL SHOW SOME DRASTIC GROWTH IN WEIGHT AND SIZE IN THIS TRIMESTER. NEAR THE END OF THE THIRD TRIMESTER YOU CAN EXPECT TO WEIGHT

25 – 35 POUNDS MORE THAN YOU HAD BEFORE YOU WERE PREGNANT. MOST OF THIS WEIGHT IS ACCOUNTED FOR THE BABY, BUT OTHER REASONS ARE ENLARGED BREASTS, AMNIOTIC FLUIDS AND EXTRA FAT.

YOU MAY NOT BE ABLE TO EAT A FULL MEAL AT A TIME BECAUSE YOUR STOMACH IS BEING PRESSED BY THE ENLARGED UTERUS, SO YOU CAN DIVIDE IT INTO SMALLER MEALS. YOU NEED TO EAT FOOD THAT WILL BOOST YOUR ENERGY AND PROVIDE AT LEAST 1,000 MG OF CALCIUM EVERY DAY. ENERGY BOOSTING FOOD CAN BE FRUITS, CHEESE, BAKED BEANS, PEANUT BUTTER, ETC.

VITAMIN K IS IMPORTANT FOR THE BIRTHING OF YOUR CHILD AND BREASTFEEDING. IT HELPS THE BLOOD TO CLOT. EXAMPLES OF VITAMIN K RICH FOODS ARE WATERCRESS, MELON, WHOLEMEAL BREAD, GREEN BEANS, WHOLEGRAIN AND BROCCOLI.

SINCE, YOU WILL BE ABLE TO MOVE AROUND LESS, YOU WILL BE MORE PRONE TO INDIGESTION. THEREFORE, CUT BACK ON COFFEE AND SPICY FOOD. SNACKING CAN HELP AS YOU WILL NEED AN EXTRA 200 CALORIES EVERY DAY DURING THIS TRIMESTER.

YOU NEED MORE ENERGY IN THE THIRD TRIMESTER TO KEEP UP WITH YOUR BODY. THE BABY GROWING INSIDE OF YOU NEEDS PLENTY OF NUTRITION AS WELL. IT MAY BECOME DIFFICULT TO DIGEST THREE WHOLE MEALS IN A DAY, WHICH IS WHY HEALTHY SNACKING IN BETWEEN MEALS IS RECOMMENDED. HERE ARE MEAL PLANS TO GET YOU THROUGH THE LAST TRIMESTER OF YOUR PREGNANCY:

SEVENTH MONTH

MEALS Days	BREAKFAST	MORNING SNACK	LUNCH	EVENING SNACK	DINNER
MONDAY	1 GLASS APPLE JUICE PORRIDGE MADE IN MILK WITH 1 TBSP APPLE	1 SMALL ROLL WITH PEANUT BUTTER.	1 SATSUMA COUSCOUS AND EGG SALAD WITH	HUMMUS WITH CARROT STICKS.	SMOKED MACKEREL PASTA WITH BABY SPINACH.

	PUREE AND A PINCH OF CINNAMON.		CURRANTS AND PINE NUTS.		
TUESDAY	A PAPAYA SMOOTHIE FROMAGE FRAIS MIXED WITH FRESH FRUITS AND 1 TBSP FLAKED ALMONDS. SERVE IT ON SCOTCH PANCAKES.	1 MUFFIN WITH 1 SLICE OF EDAM CHEESE.	A SMALL BUNCH OF GRAPES ROAST BEEF IN A BAGUETTE WITH ROCKET.	1 THICK SLICE OF BANANA BREAD.	CREAMY CURRY OF CHICK PEAS.
WEDNESDAY	1 GLASS APPLE JUICE	YOGHURT WITH	A BOWL OF MELON.	RYE CRACKERS WITH	CHICKEN RISOTT

	WHEAT CEREAL, SKIMMED MILK AND SLICED BANANAS.	BLUEBERRIES AND MELON.	BEETROOT SOUP.	SARDINE PASTE.	O.
THURSDAY	1 CUP OF HERBAL TEA PORRIDGE MADE IN MILK WITH 1 TBSP OF TINNEDBERRIES.	1 THICK SLICE OF A FRUITED MALT LOAF.	1 SLICED MANGO PITA WITH LAMB'S LETTUCE, GRUYERE AND GRAPES.	2 OR 3 MINI FALAFELS.	CREAMY FISH PIE OF HADDOCK AND SALMON WITH GREEN BEANS.
FRIDAY	A YOGHURT DRINK WHOLEGRAIN TOAST WITH SMOOTH PEANUT	2 HANDFULS OF DRIED FRUITS, INCLUDING WALNU	1 APPLE SALAD OF WATERCRESS AND SALMON.	FRUITY FLAPJACKS.	LAMB CHOPS WITH MANGETOUT AND SWEET POTAT

	BUTTER.	TS.			O WEDGES.
SATURDAY	1 GLASS ORANGE JUICE. GREEK YOGHURT WITH A TBSP OF DRIED FRUITS AND MUESLI.	A RICE POT.	1 PEAR TOASTED HAM AND CHEESE SANDWICH.	WHOLE MEAL TOAST TOPPED WITH BAKED BEANS.	BEEF LASAGNA MADE WITH SAUCE FROM RAGU AND SALAD ON THE SIDE.
SUNDAY	A YOGHURT DRINK SCRAMBLED EGGS ON A TOASTED BAGEL.	1 GLASS OF STRAWBERRY MILKSHAKE.	ROASTED LAMB, GREEN BEANS AND CARROTS.	CHEESE ON WHOLEGRAIN TOAST.	A QUICHE OF CHEESE AND SPINACH.

Eighth Month

Meals / Days	Breakfast	Morning Snack	Lunch	Evening Snack	Dinner
Monday	Apple juice. Porridge made in milk with 1 tbsp of sultanas 1 wholemeal toast with peanut butter.	Melon and blueberries with yoghurt.	1 kiwi. Beetroot soup, a crusty whole grain roll on the side.	1 cheese scone.	Creamy curry of chickpeas with rice.
Tuesday	1 strawberry milksh	Hummus with pita	1 orange. Cousco	Rye crackers spread with	Creamy fish pie of salmon,

90

	AKE. WHOLE MEAL TOAST WITH PEANUT BUTTER AND SLICED BANANAS.	BREAD.	US AND EGG SALAD, WITH CURRANTS AND PINE NUTS.	LOW FAT CHEESE.	HADDOCK, SWEETCORN AND PEAS.
WEDNESDAY	ORANGE JUICE WHEAT CEREAL, MIXED BERRY COMPOTE AND GREEK YOGHURT WITH 2 SCOTCH PANCAK	OAT, ORANGE AND CRANBERRY COOKIE.	1 BOWL OF CHOPPED MELON. TUNA SALAD WRAP.	FRUITY FLAPJACKS.	PASTA TUBES WITH SPINACH, RICOTTA AND RAGU SAUCE.

	ES.				
THURSDAY	1 CUP HERBAL TEA. FROMAGE FRAIS, 1 TBSP OF TINNED BERRIES. TOASTED TEACAKE.	WHOLEMEAL BREAD WITH PEANUT BUTTER.	1 APPLE. SOFT CHEESE AND SMOKED SALMON BAGEL.	HUMMUS WITH PITA BREAD.	CHICKEN STIR FRY NOODLES.
FRIDAY	1 YOGHURT DRINK. PORRIDGE IN MILK WITH SLICED BANANA	RICE POT	1 PEAR. BAKED POTATOES WITH CHILI.	1 SLICE OF GINGERBREAD.	SWEET APPLE LAMB, MASHED POTATOES, CARROTS AND GREEN BEANS.

	S.				
SATURDAY	ORANGE JUICE. SCRAMBLED EGGS AND A WHOLEMEAL TOAST.	FRUITY FLAPJACKS.	CHEESE AND CAULIFLOWER PASTA WITH FRUIT SALAD.	2 HOLEMEAL TOASTS WITH BAKED BEANS.	GRILLED BEEF STEAK AND BROCCOLI WITH BUTTERNUT SQUASH AND SWEET POTATO MASH.
SUNDAY	1 YOGHURT DRINK. SCOTCH PANCAKES WITH BLUEBERRIES.	1 PAPAYA SMOOTHIE WITH AN APPLE AND BRAN MUFFIN	ROASTED GAMMON, POTATOES, MANGE TOUT.	CHEESE ON WHOLEGRAIN TOAST.	A QUICHE OF CHEESE AND SPINACH WITH SALAD.

Ninth Month

MEALS Days	BREAKFAST	MORNING SNACK	LUNCH	EVENING SNACK	DINNER
MONDAY	APPLE JUICE. PORRIDGE MADE IN MILK WITH 1 TBSP OF SULTANAS. 1 WHOLEMEAL TOAST WITH PEANUT BUTTER.	MELON AND BLUEBERRIES WITH YOGHURT.	BEETROOT SOUP WITH A CRUSTY WHOLEGRAIN ROLL WITH SPREAD KIWI FRUIT	1 FRUIT SCONE.	CREAMY CURRY OF CHICKPEAS WITH RICE.
TUESDAY	1 STRAWBERRY	HUMMUS WITH	1 ORANGE. COUSCO	RYE CRACKERS SPREAD	CREAMY FISH PIE OF

	MILKSHAKE. WHOLEMEAL TOAST WITH PEANUT BUTTER AND SLICED BANANAS.	PITA BREAD.	US AND EGG SALAD, WITH CURRANTS AND PINE NUTS.	WITH LOW FAT CHEESE.	SALMON, HADDOCK, SWEETCORN AND PEAS.
WEDNESDAY	ORANGE JUICE. WHEAT CEREAL, MIXED BERRY COMPOTE AND GREEK YOGHURT WITH 2 SCOTCH	OAT, ORANGE AND CRANBERRY COOKIE.	1 BOWL OF CHOPPED MELON. TUNA SALAD WRAP.	FRUITY FLAPJACKS.	PASTA TUBES WITH SPINACH, RICOTTA AND RAGU SAUCE.

	PANCAKES.				
THURSDAY	1 CUP HERBAL TEA. FROMAGE FRAIS, 1 TBSP OF TINNED BERRIES. TOASTED TEACAKE.	WHOLEMEAL BREAD WITH PEANUT BUTTER AND A RICE POT.	1 APPLE. SARDINES ON TOAST.	HUMMUS WITH PITA BREAD.	LAMB AND MUSHROOM CASSEROLE.
FRIDAY	1 YOGHURT DRINK. PORRIDGE IN MILK WITH SLICED BANANA	FRUITY FLAPJACKS	1 PEAR. BAKED POTATOES WITH CHILI.	1 SLICE OF GINGERBREAD.	GRILLED PORK CHOPS WITH MASHED POTATOES, CARROTS AND

	S.				GREEN BEANS.
SATURDAY	ORANGE JUICE. SCRAMBLED EGGS AND A WHOLEMEAL TOAST.	1 PAPAYA SMOOTHIE. APPLE AND BRAN MUFFIN.	CHEESE AND CAULIFLOWER PASTA WITH FRUIT SALAD.	WHOLEMEAL TOAST WITH BAKED BEANS.	GRILLED BEEF STEAK AND BROCCOLI WITH BUTTERNUT SQUASH AND SWEET POTATO MASH.
SUNDAY	1 YOGHURT DRINK. SCOTCH PANCAKES WITH BLUEBERRIES.	2 HANDFULS OF DRIED FRUITS.	ROASTED CHICKEN, POTATOES, MANGE TOUT	CHEESE ON WHOLEGRAIN TOAST.	A QUICHE OF CHEESE AND SPINACH WITH SALAD.

Exercising While Pregnant

N O DIET PLAN CAN WORK WITHOUT THE APPROPRIATE EXERCISE. THE SAME IS TRUE FOR A PREGNANCY DIET PLAN. CONTRARY TO POPULAR BELIEF, EXERCISING DURING PREGNANCY CAN ALSO HELP YOU COPE BETTER WITH THE PHYSICAL AND MENTAL CHANGES YOU ARE EXPERIENCING. EXERCISE IS 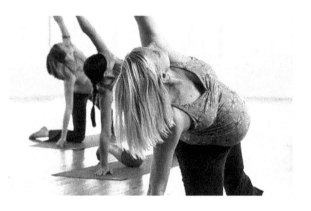 ESSENTIAL FOR A HEALTHY PREGNANCY. DURING PREGNANCY MOST WOMEN COMMONLY SUFFER FROM FATIGUE, BACKACHE AND CONSTIPATION. AN EFFECTIVE EXERCISE ROUTINE CAN HELP YOU KEEP THESE NIGGLES AT BAY. YOUR BACK IS STRENGTHENED AND THERE ARE LESS BACKACHES. IT CAN ALSO HELP YOU AVOID DEVELOPING PROBLEMS LIKE GESTATIONAL DIABETES OR PRE-ECLAMPSIA.

The most obvious benefit of exercising during pregnancy is that it will help you keep a firm hand on the weight gain. You won't gain excessive weight and you baby will receive maximum nutrients.

Also, physical exercise releases endorphins in your body that generally lift your mood. You will have less mood swings and your partner will be more than happy about it.

Many women find it hard to sleep at night during pregnancy, which results in even more fatigue. After a workout in the day, you will be so exhausted at night that you will easily fall asleep.

Exercise makes the body stronger. This will also help your body prepare for time of child birth.

SOME PRECAUTIONS

THE BEST FORM OF EXERCISE DURING PREGNANCY IS ONE THAT FULFILLS THESE CONDITIONS:

 KEEPS YOU FIT.

 HELPS YOU MANAGE WEIGHT.

 GETS YOUR HEART PUMPING.

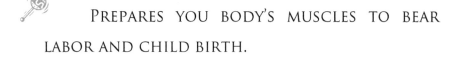 PREPARES YOU BODY'S MUSCLES TO BEAR LABOR AND CHILD BIRTH.

DOES NOT CAUSE ANY SORT OF STRESS ON YOU OR YOUR BABY.

AVOID FORMS OF EXERCISE IN WHICH YOU MAY BE AT THE RISK OF FALLING DOWN HARD OR LOSING BALANCE. EXAMPLES OF THESE TYPES OF EXERCISES ARE SKIING, FOOTBALL, TENNIS, GYMNASTICS AND HORSE-RIDING.

BEFORE UNDERTAKING ANY TYPE OF EXERCISE DURING PREGNANCY, MAKE SURE THAT YOU CONSULT YOUR OBSTETRICIAN/GYNECOLOGIST AND ONLY DO THE TYPE OF EXERCISE THAT IS SUITABLE FOR YOUR CONDITION.

BEST FORMS OF EXERCISE IN PREGNANCY

ALL EXERCISE ROUTINES NEED TO BE ALTERED AS YOUR PREGNANCY PROGRESSES. STRESSFUL EXERCISE IS NOT PRESCRIBED IN THE BEGINNING OF THE PREGNANCY BECAUSE YOU BODY IS STILL ADAPTING TO CHANGE AND YOU NEED MORE REST.

LOW OR NO-IMPACT EXERCISE IS IDEAL WHILE YOU ARE PREGNANT, SINCE IT IS EASIEST ON YOUR JOINTS. DON'T FORGET THAT ANY EXERCISE THAT DOESN'T REQUIRE YOU TO TRY TO MAINTAIN YOUR BALANCE OVER UNEVEN OR SLIPPERY GROUND IS BEST.

THE MAIN GOAL OF EXERCISING THROUGH PREGNANCY IS TO STRENGTHEN YOUR MUSCLES, IMPROVE YOUR CIRCULATION, EASE ANY BACKACHE, AND HELP YOU FEEL WELL. IT'S IMPORTANT TO AVOID ANY EXERCISE OR ACTIVITIES THAT REQUIRE JUMPY AND JERKY MOVEMENTS, TAKE SHARP CHANGES OF DIRECTION, OR IS SO VIGOROUS THAT IT RAISES YOUR CORE TEMPERATURE OR PUTS EXCESSIVE STRAIN ON YOUR CARDIOVASCULAR SYSTEM OR JOINTS.

IN ADDITION, IMPACT SPORTS AND SPORTS THAT INVOLVE A RISK OF FALLING, SUCH AS CYCLING, HORSE

RIDING, DOWNHILL SKIING, AND CONTACT SPORTS ARE NOT ADVISABLE.

SOME GOOD CHOICES ARE LISTED BELOW.

Walking, Jogging or Running

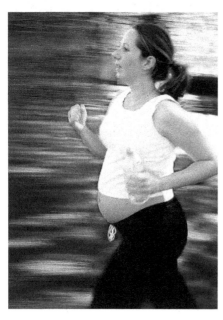

WALKING PROVIDES YOU AN EXCELLENT CARDIO WORKOUT WITHOUT PUTTING YOU AT ANY KIND OF RISK. IT IS ALSO COMPLETELY SAFE THROUGH YOUR ENTIRE PREGNANCY. YOU CAN INCORPORATE IT INTO YOUR DAILY ROUTINE. EVEN IF YOU ARE UNABLE TO GET ANY OTHER FORM OF EXERCISE, YOU CAN ALWAYS GO FOR A WALK. JOGGING AND RUNNING ARE THE MOST EFFICIENT WAYS TO GET A GOOD WORKOUT TO GET YOUR HEART PUMPING. HOWEVER, IF YOU WERE NOT A JOGGER OR RUNNER BEFORE YOU GOT PREGNANT, IT IS NOT THE RIGHT TIME TO START IT NOW. GO FOR A WALK INSTEAD.

SWIMMING AND WALKING ARE THE SAFEST FORMS OF EXERCISE DURING PREGNANCY. SWIMMING LETS YOU EXERCISE YOUR MUSCLES AND GETS YOUR HEART PUMPING. IT IS SAFE TO CARRY OUT

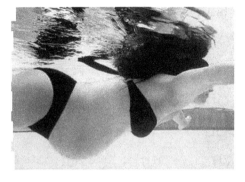

SWIMMING THROUGHOUT YOUR PREGNANCY.

AQUANATAL

AQUANATAL CLASSES HAVE ALSO BECOME VERY POPULAR

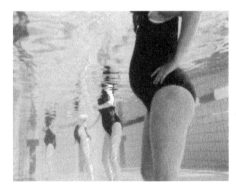

LATELY. YOU MAY WANT TO CONSIDER JOINING ONE OF THOSE IF YOU DON'T .LIKE TO SWIM ALONE. EXERCISE ROUTINES IN AQUANATAL CLASSES ARE GOOD FOR THE JOINTS AND CAN ALSO HELP EASE THE SWELLING FROM YOUR FEET AND LEGS.

PILATES

THIS FORM OF EXERCISE HELPS YOU STRENGTHEN YOU PELVIC FLOOR MUSCLES AND TUMMY. PILATES CLASSES FOR PREGNANT WOMEN INCLUDE EXERCISE ROUTINES THAT ARE SAFE FOR YOUR CONDITION.

YOU INSTRUCTOR WILL GUIDE YOU THROUGH A SERIES OF PHYSICAL AND BREATHING EXERCISES

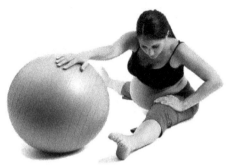

THAT WILL HELP YOU RELAX YOUR MIND AND BODY. THIS WILL HELP YOU WITH BREATHING IN LABOR AT THE TIME OF CHILD BIRTH. IT IS SAFE TO CARRY OUT AS LONG AS YOU CAN IN YOUR PREGNANCY.

YOGA

WOMEN ENDURE A LOT OF PHYSICAL AND EMOTIONAL STRESS DURING PREGNANCY. WITHOUT ATTAINING RELIEF, YOUR BODY MAY NOT BE ABLE TO HANDLE PREGNANCY, PHYSICALLY AND ESPECIALLY EMOTIONALLY.

YOGA IS INCREDIBLY BENEFICIAL FOR PREGNANT WOMEN. AS YOU KNOW, YOU NEED TO RELAX YOUR BODY, CALM YOUR MIND AND BREATHE DEEPLY DURING YOGA POSES. THIS CAN HELP REDUCE THE PHYSICAL

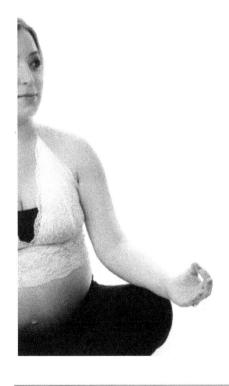

STRAIN ON THE BODY AND CAN HELP SIGNIFICANTLY DURING LABOR.

IF YOU TAKE YOGA CLASSES ON A REGULAR BASIS, JUST REMEMBER TO LET YOUR INSTRUCTOR KNOW THAT YOU ARE PREGNANT. ALSO, ENSURE THAT THEY KNOW WHICH TRIMESTER YOU ARE IN. THAT WILL GIVE THEM AN IDEA OF WHAT

EXERCISES ARE GOOD FOR YOU.

IF YOU ARE DOING YOGA FOR THE FIRST TIME, IT IS A GOOD IDEA TO JOIN PRENATAL YOGA CLASSES. ADDITIONALLY, CONTACT YOUR DOCTOR AND MAKE SURE YOGA IS SAFE FOR YOU.

WEIGHT TRAINING

IF YOU ARE AN ACTIVE WOMAN, YOU PROBABLY PERFORM WEIGHT-TRAINING EXERCISES AT LEAST 3-4 TIMES A WEEK. IT HELPS IMPROVE YOUR MUSCLES AND IMPROVES BLOOD 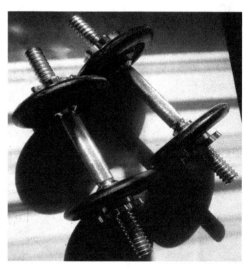 CIRCULATION. IT ALSO KEEPS THE BODY TONED.

UNFORTUNATELY, AS A PREGNANT WOMAN, THERE WILL BE A FEW RESTRICTIONS PLACED ON YOUR WEIGHT-TRAINING EXERCISES. THERE WILL BE CASES WHERE YOU CANNOT PERFORM CERTAIN EXERCISES.

THERE WILL ALSO BE TIMES WHEN YOU CANNOT LIFT THE SAME WEIGHTS YOU USED TO. FOR ONE, YOU

CANNOT LIFT HEAVY WEIGHTS AS THIS COULD CAUSE YOUR CHILD HARM. INSTEAD, TRY USING HALF THE WEIGHTS YOU USED TO LIFT AND INCREASE THE REPETITIONS.

YOU CANNOT LIE DOWN AND DO BENCH PRESSES ANYMORE AS IT REDUCES THE AMOUNT OF BLOOD GOING TO YOUR CHILD; IT IS DETRIMENTAL IF DONE TOO OFTEN OR FOR TOO LONG. IF YOU STILL NEED TO DO YOUR CHEST EXERCISES, DO THEM ON AN INCLINED BENCH. THIS SIGNIFICANTLY REDUCES THE RISK TO YOU AND YOUR CHILD.

ONE OF THE WORST THINGS YOU CAN DO IS BRING YOUR DUMBBELLS CLOSE TO YOUR ABDOMEN. MANY EXERCISES REQUIRE THAT YOU BRING THE DUMBBELLS CLOSE TO YOUR ABDOMEN. IN FACT, THERE ARE MANY EXERCISES IN WHICH THAT HAPPENS NATURALLY. YOU NEED TO AVOID THESE EXERCISES AS THEY CAN HARM YOUR CHILD.

ALTHOUGH WALKING LUNGES ARE GREAT FOR YOUR LEGS AND PELVIC MUSCLES, IT IS DANGEROUS DURING PREGNANCY. THE LAST THING YOU WANT IS DAMAGED PELVIC MUSCLES DURING LABOR.

BEFORE PERFORMING ANY WEIGHT TRAINING EXERCISE, MAKE SURE YOU CONSULT WITH YOUR DOCTOR FIRST.

CYCLING

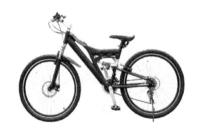 AT FIRST, YOU MAY THINK THAT CYCLING IS THE LAST THING YOU WOULD WANT TO DO WHEN YOU ARE PREGNANT. THE SEAT WILL FEEL UNCOMFORTABLE, THE BUMPS CAN HURT YOU AND YOUR CHILD AND THEN THERE IS THE DANGER OF FALLING. HOWEVER, MOST OF THESE DANGERS EXIST WHEN YOU ARE DRIVING A CAR AS WELL. IF YOU ARE A FREQUENT BIKE RIDER, THERE IS ABSOLUTELY NO PROBLEM IF YOU RIDE YOUR BIKE EVERY NOW AND AGAIN. JUST MAKE SURE THAT YOUR SEAT IS WELL PADDED AND PROPERLY ANGLED. FURTHERMORE, ENSURE THAT YOU DO NOT RIDE UPHILL, IN GROUPS OR ON THE MAIN ROAD AS THIS CAN INCREASE THE CHANCES THAT YOU FALL OFF YOUR BIKE.

WHEN PREGNANT, RIDING YOUR BIKE CAN BE ONE OF THE MOST RELAXING THINGS YOU CAN DO. IT HELPS STRENGTHEN YOUR MUSCLES, IMPROVES YOUR BREATHING AND HELPS RELAX THE BODY. YOU ALSO GET A CHANCE TO ENJOY THE OUTDOORS. THE COMBINED EFFECTS HELP TO ALLEVIATE EMOTIONAL STRESS.

Do's & Don'ts for Diabetic Pregnant Women

Being diabeticis not easy when you are pregnant. A pregnancy where the expecting mom is diabetic is termed as a high-risk pregnancy. Fortunately, in no way does this mean that you won't have a healthy baby. It simply means that you need to watch out for more things than regular pregnant women.

Regardless of whether you have been diagnosed with Type 1 or Type 2 diabetes, it is important that you understand a few do's and don'ts. They will ensure that your pregnancy goes smoothly and that you give birth to a healthy baby.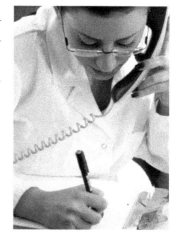

Being diabetic is not a cause for alarm. You don't need to worry about a million and one things. In fact, the ensuing stress of doing so will prove problematic for both you and your baby.

Millions of diabetic women become pregnant and give birth to healthy babies without causing problems for the mom. All you need to do is keep a few things in mind and you will be fine. In other words, simply follow the do's and don'ts outlined below and I promise you will have a happy and healthy pregnancy.

Do's

Talking to a gynecologist or an obstetrician is the obvious choice for pregnant women. In fact, it is the smart choice. However, when you have diabetes, it is an even better idea to talk to a perinatologist.

Perinatologists are your normal gynecologists and/or obstetricians who have completed further training, specializing in high-risk pregnancies. This also includes diabetic pregnancies.

Eat in Moderation

Although this really does go without saying, as a diabetic, it is even more crucial to eat in moderation. As a diabetic, you need to maintain your blood glucose level all day long. If your blood glucose level drops or increases too much, it could prove harmful for you. However, when you are pregnant, it could harm your baby too.

Your baby's only supply of glucose comes directly from your own supply. If you do not have enough glucose to spare, your baby will not be able to grow properly.

If you have a high blood glucose level, you can 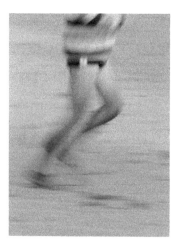 experience a varied number of problems. However, your child can experience more, with the biggest problem being obesity. A high blood glucose level increases the risk of bearing an obese child. This can prove highly problematic for many women during labor.

EXERCISE

One of the biggest mistakes that most pregnant women make is avoiding exercise. Not only does this lead to a higher postpartum weight, it could also result in an obese baby. During a diabetic pregnancy, not exercising is the worst thing you can do.

The only 2 ways to really keep your blood sugar levels down is by either exercise or insulin. Considering the many advantages that exercise has, it makes sense to choose it over the injections.

However, make sure you visit your health care provider and get an exercise plan made. The last thing you need to do is exercise too much as this will significantly lower your blood glucose levels.

Don'ts

Snack on Sweets of any Kind

The worst thing you could actually do during your pregnancy is snack on a multitude of sweets. Not only does this raise your blood glucose level, it

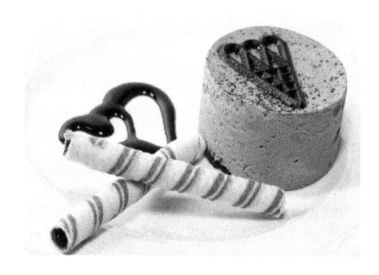

adds empty calories to your body.

If you have diabetes, you need to pay close attention to the food you eat in terms of the amount of sugar they contain.

Keep your Carbohydrates Down

During pregnancy, the first thing that most health care providers will recommend is that

YOU KEEP YOUR STRENGTH UP BY CONSUMING A LOT OF CARBOHYDRATES. UNFORTUNATELY, CARBOHYDRATE IS A MOLECULE THAT EASILY TURNS INTO GLUCOSE. THIS BECOMES A DIABETIC'S WORST NIGHTMARE. TO OVERCOME THIS ISSUE, THE EASIEST THING TO DO IS PLAN YOUR MEALS.

THE KEY IS TO CONTROL THE AMOUNT OF CARBOHYDRATES THAT YOU CONSUME DOWN TO A MINIMUM. THOUGH, KNOWING THE AMOUNT OF CARBOHYDRATES YOU SHOULD CONSUME IS SOMETHING THAT ONLY YOUR DOCTOR CAN ACCURATELY TELL YOU AS THEY KNOW ABOUT YOUR CONDITION AND MEDICAL HISTORY.

THEY WILL BE ABLE TO TELL YOU, ROUGHLY, HOW MANY CARBS YOU SHOULD CONSUME EVERY DAY. THEY WILL ALSO LET YOU KNOW OF ANY SPECIAL DIETS THAT YOU SHOULD BE ON. THIS INFORMATION SHOULD BE TAKEN TO A DIETICIAN IN ORDER TO OBTAIN A PROPER DIET PLAN.

SKIP A MEAL

IF YOU ARE DIABETIC, AND ARE PREGNANT, THE WORST THING YOU COULD DO FOR YOURSELF IS SKIP A MEAL.

BREAKFAST IS THE MOST IMPORTANT MEAL OF THE DAY AND BY SKIPPING IT, YOU LOWER YOUR BLOOD GLUCOSE LEVELS SIGNIFICANTLY. NOT ONLY DOES THIS ENSURE YOU HAVE NO ENERGY FOR THE DAY, IT CAN BE HARMFUL FOR YOUR BABY TOO.

EXERCISE TOO MUCH

EXERCISE IS A GREAT WAY TO LET LOOSE, LOSE A POUND OR TWO AND MAINTAIN A HEALTHY LIFESTYLE. WHEN YOU ARE A PREGNANT, YOU SHOULD EXERCISE IN ORDER TO KEEP YOUR MOOD ELEVATED AND YOUR BODY AND CHILD HAPPY.

HOWEVER, TOO MUCH EXERCISE AND YOU RISK LOWERING YOUR BLOOD GLUCOSE LEVEL TOO MUCH, CAUSING WEAKNESS, MENTAL DISTURBANCES, EMOTIONAL FRUSTRATION AND POSSIBLY PHYSICAL COLLAPSE. THEREFORE, NEVER EXERCISE MORE THAN YOU HAVE TO.

Post Partum

The first few hours, days, and weeks with a newborn can be challenging, but delightful at the same time. This chapter will prepare you for what to expect. Read up on breast- feeding and bottle-feeding so you're ready to go as soon as your baby is. Once you finally have your beautiful new baby to cuddle and love, information on practical baby care will help you get the best out of your precious time together.

SKIN-TO-SKIN CONTACT

One hour of skin-to-skin contact immediately after birth makes a baby significantly less stressed after the trauma of the birth experience.

During skin-to-skin contact, your baby's heartbeat and breathing are more regular and stable.

Babies who have regular skin-to-skin contact tend to cry less.

BABIES WHO HAVE SKIN-TO-SKIN CONTACT DIGEST THEIR FOOD BETTER.

98.6° F (37.5° C) IS THE NORMAL BODY TEMPERATURE. DURING SKIN-TO-SKIN CONTACT YOUR BODY HELPS TO REGULATE YOUR BABY'S TEMPERATURE AND KEEP IT AT THE RIGHT LEVEL.

SKIN-TO-SKIN CONTACT HELPS YOUR BABY PICK UP FRIENDLY BACTERIA FROM YOUR SKIN, WHICH PROTECT HER FROM CATCHING INFECTIONS.

SKIN-TO-SKIN CONTACT HELPS ESTABLISH BREAST-FEEDING BECAUSE YOUR BABY CAN SEE AND SMELL THE NIPPLE, WHICH ENCOURAGES HER TO FEED.

SKIN-TO-SKIN CONTACT HELPS TRIGGER YOUR BREAST MILK TO FLOW.

SKIN-TO-SKIN CONTACT HELPS MAKE YOU FEEL MORE CONFIDENT THAT YOU CAN TAKE CARE OF YOUR BABY.

Breast Feeding

BREASTFEEDING IS THE ACT OF A MOTHER GIVING HER CHILD MILK DIRECTLY FROM HER BREAST. THIS IS ALSO KNOWN AS LACTATION.

BABIES LATCH THEMSELVES ONTO THE MOTHER'S BREAST, AIDED BY THE MOTHER, AND SUCK THE BREAST

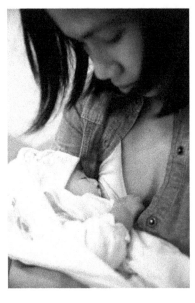 MILK. THE TRUTH IS THAT THERE IS NO BETTER MILK FOR A CHILD THAN BREAST MILK. BREAST MILK SHOULD BE GIVEN TO THE BABY FOR AT LEAST 6 MONTHS. THE MOTHER CAN CONTINUE FOR A YEAR IF SHE DESIRES.

HEALTH ORGANIZATIONS, SUCH AS THE AMERICAN ACADEMY OF PEDIATRICS (APP) RECOMMEND THAT MOTHERS CONTINUE SUPPLEMENTAL BREASTFEEDING FOR AT LEAST A YEAR AFTER THE FIRST 6 MONTHS. HOWEVER, THE WORLD HEALTH ORGANIZATION (WHO) RECOMMENDS A PERIOD OF 2 YEARS.

BREAST-FEEDING COMMON CONCERNS

UNDERSTANDING THE CAUSES OF BREAST-FEEDING DISCOMFORTS CAN HELP PREVENT THEM FROM BECOMING WORSE. TAKE ACTION AS SOON AS POSSIBLE TO RESOLVE ANY PROBLEMS SO THAT EFFICIENT FEEDING CAN BE ESTABLISHED.

Sore, cracked, and bleeding nipples

It's normal for your nipples to feel tender since your baby's sucking stretches them, but sore nipples that last beyond the first week can indicate a problem that needs addressing. If the nipples become cracked, you may experience sharp pain for a few seconds at the beginning of a feeding. Cracked nipples may also bleed, and your baby may swallow some blood. Streaks of blood may appear in your baby's stools or when he spits up. Although alarming, this isn't harmful for your baby.

CAUSES: If your baby isn't latched on correctly, he may suck on your nipple, rather than your breast tissue. This makes the nipple increasingly tender, and the pressure of the sucking can cause the nipple to crack, and sometimes bleed. Since your nipples are often moist when breast-feeding, it is hard for the cracks to heal. If nipples suddenly become red and sore after a period of being fine, you may have thrush, a fungal infection that can pass between you and your baby. You will both need medical care.

Blocked milk duct

A blocked duct can result in a lump with swelling and inflammation, and the area may be tender. The swelling may be alleviated slightly after breast-feeding. If bacteria reach the blocked duct, it can lead to mastitis.

CAUSES: Milk ducts form a series of channels that carry milk to your nipple. A milk duct can become blocked if your breast isn't drained completely, often because your baby has a poor latch or has a weak suck. In the early days, when your breasts are producing a lot of milk, they may become engorged, leading to a blocked duct. A badly fitting bra can put pressure on a part of the breast and cause a blockage. If you have redness, swelling, and lumps, contact your doctor. Early treatment can help avoid further complications, such as mastitis.

Mastitis and breast abscess

If you have hardness, swelling, and redness, and your temperature is slightly raised, you may have mastitis. If the infection worsens, it can become very painful, your temperature may

ESCALATE, AND YOU MAY HAVE FLULIKE SYMPTOMS. OCCASIONALLY, PUS FORMS IN THE AREA AND AN ABSCESS DEVELOPS, WHICH FEELS LIKE AN EXTREMELY PAINFUL LUMP. MASTITIS IS MOST COMMON IN THE EARLY WEEKS OF BREAST- FEEDING WHEN YOUR MILK SUPPLY HASN'T YET

SETTLED DOWN.

<u>CAUSES</u>: PROBLEMS CAN STEM FROM YOUR BABY HAVING A POOR LATCH OR WEAK SUCKING, WHICH LEADS TO A BLOCKED DUCT OR AN AREA WHERE THERE IS A BUILD UP OF MILK, REFERRED TO AS MILK STASIS. IF BACTERIA PRESENT ON YOUR SKIN TRAVEL TO A BLOCKED MILK DUCT, IT CAN CAUSE A MASTITIS INFECTION. IF YOU ARE ANEMIC, OR VERY RUN DOWN, YOUR RESISTANCE MAY BE LOWERED, MAKING YOU MORE SUSCEPTIBLE TO INFECTION.

CHANGES

DURING BREASTFEEDING, THE BREAST ITSELF ENLARGES AS IT FILLS WITH BREAST MILK. IN OTHER WORDS, THE BREASTS SEEM FULLER. FOR FIRST TIME MOMS, THE

NIPPLES MAY FEEL A LITTLE SORE OR TENDER AFTER THE FIRST BREASTFEEDING SESSION.

THE AREOLA (AREA AROUND THE NIPPLE) WILL ALSO ENLARGE. THE NIPPLE WILL ALSO SLIGHTLY INCREASE IN SIZE, ALLOWING THE BABY TO EASILY LATCH ONTO THE NIPPLE AND SUCK THE BREAST MILK.

HOW TO BREAST FEED YOUR CHILD

FOR NEW MOMS, IT IS A GOOD IDEA TO LATCH THE BABY IN A CRADLE POSITION. YOU SHOULD BRING THE BABY TO YOUR NIPPLE RATHER THAN THE OPPOSITE. IT IS A GOOD IDEA TO PUT A PILLOW UNDER THE BABY TO SUPPORT HIS/HER WEIGHT. REMEMBER THAT YOUR CHILD CAN BREAST FEED FOR ANYWHERE BETWEEN 5 MINUTES AND AN HOUR.

IN MANY CASES, THE NIPPLES OF NEW MOMS WILL FEEL A LITTLE SORE AFTER A BREASTFEEDING SESSION. THIS IS NORMAL. HOWEVER, IF IT FEELS THIS WAY AFTER A FEW SESSIONS, IT IS HIGHLY LIKELY THAT YOU ARE NOT LATCHING YOUR BABY PROPERLY. THE EASIEST WAY AROUND IT IS TO CONSULT YOUR PRIMARY HEALTH CARE PROVIDER OR A LACTATION SPECIALIST.

Post Partum Depression

Practically every woman will experience post partum depression. Although the reason behind the cause of post partum depression is not well understood, it is thought that a hormonal change brings up the changes. Post partum depression can last up to a year.

The symptoms of post partum depression include:

- ❖ Guilt
- ❖ Sadness
- ❖ Hopelessness
- ❖ Fatigue
- ❖ Emptiness
- ❖ Sleepy
- ❖ High irritability
- ❖ Impaired motor functions
- ❖ Anxiety
- ❖ Panic attacks
- ❖ Disturbances during sleep
- ❖ Anger
- ❖ Decreased Libido

However, not every case of post partum depression is the same. Here are a few factors that affect the intensity and duration of post partum depression.

❖ Guilt over not breastfeeding the child.
❖ A long medical history of clinical depression.
❖ Smoking.
❖ Alcohol.
❖ Low self-esteem.
❖ Low social, financial and emotional support.
❖ Anxiety as a new parent.
❖ Poor marriage.
❖ Stress.
❖ The fact that the child was unplanned.

Warning signs

You find it hard to sleep, have fitful sleep, or wake too early feeling anxious.

You feel low-level anxiety, or perhaps feel very anxious and suffer from panic attacks.

You feel irritable and lack concentration.

You struggle to feel enjoyment or pleasure in life, and lack humor.

You feel guilty and generally miserable.

Your appetite is poor, or you overeat.

You feel lethargic, tired, and unmotivated, and you aren't managing to take care of yourself properly.

You feel isolated.

You have little interest in your baby.

Support

Talk to your partner, or other loved ones, and consult your doctor if you experience any of the warning signs more than a week after the birth. Don't ignore these feelings since they are easily treatable—if left they can affect your relationship with your baby, partner, and others.

If you have suffered from depression before, the symptoms will feel familiar, although with PPD there is the added factor of how your illness impacts your baby and your relationship with him. Getting help may make all the difference in your experience of motherhood.

CONCLUSION

PREGNANCY IS AN AMAZING TIME IN ANY WOMAN'S LIFE. IT IS THE TIME WHEN YOU GIVE BIRTH TO A HUMAN CHILD. FROM THE DAY YOU FIND OUT YOU ARE PREGNANT TO THE DAY YOU HOLD YOUR CHILD FOR THE FIRST TIME IN YOUR HANDS, YOU WILL ENJOY AND TREASURE EVERY MOMENT OF YOUR BEAUTIFUL JOURNEY.

THERE WILL BE TIMES WHERE YOU WILL FEEL LIKE THE HAPPIEST PERSON IN THE WORLD, AS YOU SHOULD. THERE WILL BE TIMES WHERE YOU FEEL LIKE SCREAMING AT EVERYTHING AND EVERYONE AROUND YOU. REMEMBER, YOU ARE NEVER ALONE.

ASIDE FROM ALL THE JOY, DON'T FORGET THAT YOU NEED TO CONTROL YOUR DIET THROUGHOUT THE PREGNANCY. ENSURE THAT YOUR DIET IS FULL OF A VARIETY OF FRESH AND HEALTHY FOOD. I KNOW IT WILL BE HARD TO FIGHT THE CRAVINGS BUT YOU NEED TO STAY AWAY FROM UNHEALTHY, GREASY AND FAT-FILLED FOOD.

MOST IMPORTANTLY, DO NOT FORGET THAT DAILY EXERCISE ALSO INCORPORATES A GOOD PREGNANCY

DIET. WHETHER YOU GO FOR A BRISK WALK IN THE MORNING OR PERFORM YOGA THROUGHOUT THE DAY, ENSURE THAT YOU KEEP YOUR BODY MOBILE.

BY FOLLOWING THIS GUIDE, YOU WILL HAVE A HAPPY AND HEALTHY PREGNANCY. REMEMBER, THIS GUIDE IS IN NO WAY AN ALTERNATIVE TO A CONSULTATION. IT IS A GUIDE TO HELP YOU DECIDE WHICH FOODS TO EAT DURING A PREGNANCY. ALWAYS CONSULT YOUR PRIMARY HEALTH CARE PROVIDER BEFORE STARTING ANY NEW DIET.

NOTES

CPSIA information can be obtained
at www.ICGtesting.com
Printed in the USA
BVHW091044260521
608177BV00009B/842

9 781802 853742